How to Prepare for the Praxis Examination in Speech-Language Pathology

How to Prepare for the Praxis Examination in Speech-Language Pathology

Second Edition

Kay T. Payne, Ph.D.
Department of Communication Sciences and Disorders
Howard University
Washington, D.C.

SINGULAR
THOMSON LEARNING™

Australia • Canada • Mexico • Singapore • Spain • United Kingdom • United States

WB

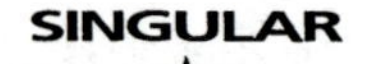

How to Prepare for the Praxis Examination in Speech-Language Pathology, Second Edition

by Kay T. Payne, Ph.D.

Business Unit Director:
William Brottmiller

Acquisitions Editor:
Marie Linvill

Editorial Assistant:
Kristin Banach

Executive Marketing Manager:
Dawn Gerrain

Channel Manager:
Tara Carter

Executive Production Manager:
Karen Leet

Production Editor:
Sandy Doyle

Printed in Canada
3 4 5 XXX 05 04 02

For more information contact Singular,
401 West "A" Street, Suite 325
San Diego, CA 92101-7904
Or find us on the World Wide Web at http://www.singpub.com

Library of Congress
Cataloging-in-Publication Data
Payne, Kay T.
How to prepare for the Praxis in speech-language pathology / by Kay T. Payne.
p. ; cm.
Updated version of: part of How to prepare for the NESPA, 1991. Companion v. to: How to prepare for the Praxis in audiology. Includes bibliographical references.
ISBN 0-7693-0160-6 (soft cover)
1. Speech Disorders—Examinations, questions, etc. 2. Language Disorders—Examinations, questions, etc. I. Payne, Kay T. How to prepare for the NESPA. II. Payne, Kay T. How to prepare for the Praxis in audiology. III. Title.
[DNLM: 1. Speech Disorders—Examination Questions. 2. Language Disorders—Examination Questions. WV 18.2 P346h 2001]
RC423 .P355 2001
616.5'5'0076—dc21 00-037162

NOTICE TO THE READER

Publisher does not warrant or guarantee any of the products described herein or perform any independent analysis in connection with any of the product information contained herein. Publisher does not assume, and expressly disclaims, any obligation to obtain and include information other than that provided to it by the manufacturer.

The reader is expressly warned to consider and adopt all safety precautions that might be indicated by the activities herein and to avoid all potential hazards. By following the instructions contained herein, the reader willingly assumes all risks in connection with such instructions.

The Publisher makes no representation or warranties of any kind, including but not limited to, the warranties of fitness for particular purpose or merchantability, nor are any such representations implied with respect to the material set forth herein, and the publisher takes no responsibility with respect to such material. The publisher shall not be liable for any special, consequential, or exemplary damages resulting, in whole or part, from the readers' use of, or reliance upon, this material.

3/4/05

CONTENTS

PREFACE

This volume—*How to Prepare for the Praxis Examination in Speech-Language Pathology*—is an updated version of *How to Prepare for the NESPA*, first published in 1991. That work was an outgrowth of research conducted at Howard University through a grant from the U.S. Department of Education. For many years, the author noted a difference in performance of minority test takers on almost any standard measure. Sensing a "cultural bias" the author endeavored to identify the source of the bias. Instead, what was found was a more prevalent "test-taker bias" that affects many individuals. This can be observed in the phenomena wherein very good students are sometimes poor standardized test takers, and inversely, mediocre students can be very good standardized test takers.

The philosophical basis of this volume is that knowledge of subject matter is but a mere fraction of what is required for success on standardized tests. A successful test-taking experience is a combination of knowledge, critical thinking, clinical judgment, reasoning ability, test-taking strategy, and quick timing. Success also depends on affective qualities such as mental outlook and confidence. Lack of any one, or a combination, of the requirements might contribute to unsuccessful performance. The author believes that successful test-taking skills can be coached and developed. Therefore, this test improves on the earlier volume by providing discussion of the necessary skills and processes for successful performance on the Praxis. Several new improvements have been made to the units.

Additions to Unit 1 include an extensive bibliography of what to study and relevant Web page addresses. The mini-examinations of Units 3, 4, 7, 8, and 9 have been revised. Unit 5 includes a new list of sight words and phrases typical of Praxis questions that will assist in increasing reading speed. A totally new Unit 6 discusses mental preparation, expanding the discussion of test anxiety and cognitive style to include both psychological and physical preparation.

Sincere gratitude is expressed to individuals without whom this book would not have been possible. Ms. Rhesa John, Ms. Kimberly Springer, and Ms. Kelly Fair, students at Howard University, provided invaluable and loyal service as research assistants. Dr. Noma Anderson lent her expertise to the previous volume, which served as the foundation to this text. There were numerous other friends, family, colleagues, and students whose informal discussions also helped to shape the concepts of this book.

It is my dream that this book will be a source of assistance to all those by whom it is needed.

For

Kenneth Evans Payne

Anna Strickland Payne

UNIT 1

STUDYING FOR THE PRAXIS

Before you begin to study for an examination as important as the Praxis, you should consider your own study habits, as well as what is required to be successful on the examination. First, assess your study habits by taking the following multiple choice test.

1. How would you describe your usual study habits in relation to your testing success?

    A. I don't have to study much to get good grades
    B. The more I study, the better my grades
    C. If I don't study, my grades suffer
    D. Even when I study, my grades are just about the same

2. How often do you feel that you have studied, but the test focused on other information?

    A. Never
    B. Rarely
    C. Sometimes
    D. Often

3. How often do you misjudge what is to be included on an examination? That is, do you ever avoid studying some material and take a chance that it will not be on the examination, but it does appear on the examination?

    A. Never
    B. Rarely
    C. Sometimes
    D. Often

4. How often do you find that you have studied as much, or more than your peers, but your grades are not comparable?

    A. Never
    B. Rarely
    C. Sometimes
    D. Often

5. On what kind of question do you perform best?
   A. Multiple choice
   B. Fill-in/True-False
   C. Matching
   D. Essay

6. On what kind of question do you perform worst?
   A. There is no difference
   B. Multiple choice
   C. True-False/Matching/Fill-in
   D. Essay

7. When you guess on an examination, how often are you correct?
   A. Almost always
   B. Usually
   C. Rarely
   D. Never

8. How often do you find that you have misinterpreted a question?
   A. Never
   B. Rarely
   C. Sometimes
   D. Often

9. How often do you feel that you know more than your test scores reflect?
   A. Never
   B. Rarely
   C. Sometimes
   D. Often

10. Are your scores on standardized tests consistent with your academic grades?
    A. Grades on standardized tests are higher than academic grades
    B. Grades on standardized tests are consistent with academic grades
    C. Grades on standardized tests are slightly lower than academic grades
    D. Grades on standardized tests are much worse than academic grades

This brief assessment can reveal much about the effectiveness of your study process. Score your test as follows. For each question:

A = 3 points
B = 2 points
C = 1 point
D = 0 points

Tally your score and interpret your study habits as listed below.

26–30 points	EXCELLENT	11–15 points	BELOW AVERAGE
21–25 points	ABOVE AVERAGE	6–10 points	POOR
16–20 points	AVERAGE	0–5 points	MISERABLE

If you had nine or more As your study habits are quite conducive to good performance on the Praxis. You probably learn very well in the classroom, thus extensive study time for the examination might not be required. Your intuitive skills for predicting what will be on the examination are also quite good. You are probably a good test-taker regardless of the types of questions presented.

If you achieved an equal combination of As and Bs your study skills are above average. You probably perform well despite a few qualities that are less than optimal. Note the consistencies in your answers: i.e., whether they lie in amount of study time, types of questions, or judgment of the content of the examination. With this knowledge the quality of your study experience can be improved.

If you achieved a preponderance of Bs and Cs your study skills are at risk. You are an Average to Below Average test taker. You should be acutely aware that effective studying is a matter of *process*, as well as content and time. Practicing the types of questions that will appear on the Praxis is the most effective study process. In addition, it is helpful to know and understand as much about the examination as possible. Part of your preparation should be reading all information presented in the bulletin of information that is available from Educational Testing Service (ETS).

In addition, you must tailor your study not only for the specific content areas of the test, but also to your individual weaknesses whether in the amount of time given to study, study procedures, or practice for the types of questions. If you are usually wrong when you guess, you must practice to improve your intuitive ability. Do this by analyzing your logic as compared to the explanation given for the correct answer in the Practice Test in the appendix. Your study should be designed to compensate for your individual weaknesses.

If your answers were mostly Cs and Ds you are at high risk for poor performance on the Praxis. Bear in mind that you may know the coursework extremely well, but for some reason your test performance is not good.

If your answers to questions 5 and 6 suggest that you are not adept at taking multiple-choice tests, perhaps the reason relates to your decision-making ability. Often the presence of more than one plausible response creates confusion. To lessen this confusion you will need to use your internal powers of concentration, reasoning, and confidence. These powers are perfected through continued practice with the Practice Test in Appendix B.

WHAT TO STUDY

Since you now know that effective studying is more a matter of process than content, you may still feel that some review of coursework is necessary. Review of coursework is especially recommended if you completed your academic study more than 1 year prior to taking the Praxis. It is important to note, however, that successful performance on the Praxis is enhanced more by your skills of *clinical judgment, critical thinking, test-taking strategies, timing,* and *effective guessing.* While many questions require the "textbook answer," most questions are presented as clinical scenarios for which direct knowledge of coursework is abstracted.

In some cases, good test takers—i.e., those who are able to utilize these five skills—perform well even without coursework knowledge. For most students, however, it is a wise choice to practice the requisite skills, as well as have knowledge of the field.

A bibliography of current resources follows which can be useful for preparation for the Praxis. For general knowledge almost any comprehensive, introductory text can be useful. For in-depth review of specific areas of coursework, a text related specifically to the content area may be necessary. Many textbooks provide an Instructor's Manual that contains summary outlines and useful test questions for practice.

TEST PREPARATION MATERIALS

Software

- Payne, K., & Tishman, A. (2000). Computer Practice Module for the Praxis Examination. San Diego, CA: Singular Publishing Group. www.singpub.com.

Multiple choice questions with 27 exercises to simulate the Praxis. Improves timing and test-taking skills. Provides computer-aided instruction and practice in each area of coursework.

Audiotape

- Nye, C. (1998). *Review course for the N.E.S.P.A.* [Audiotape]. San Diego, CA: Singular Publishing Group. www.singpub.com.

Thorough review of all subject areas. Lectures on 10 audiotapes. Serves as a confidence builder.

Study Guides

- Educational Testing Service. (1995). *A guide to the NTE Speech-Language Pathology Specialty Area Test.* Princeton, NJ: Author.

An actual Praxis test along with answers and comprehensive explanations. Contact: The Praxis Series, ETS, P.O. Box 6058, Princeton, NJ. (800) 537-3161.

- Roseberry-McKibbin, C., & Hegde, M. N. (1999). *An advanced review of speech-language pathology: Preparation for NESPA and Comprehensive Examination.* Austin, TX: Pro-Ed. www.proedinc.com.

Review outline of all areas of coursework as well as test questions and study tips.

Review Course

- National Black Association for Speech, Language and Hearing Review Course in Preparation for the National Examination in Speech-Language Pathology, Washington, DC.

Three-day intensive review of coursework and presentation of test-taking skills. Contact: NESPA Review Course, P.O. Box 50605, Washington, DC 20091-0605. NBASLH@aol.com.

Review Book

- Culbertson, W. (1999). *Study guide for human communication disorders.* Needham Heights, MA: Allyn & Bacon. www.abacon.com.

Chapter outlines, summaries, essay, true/false and multiple-choice questions and answers.

GENERAL TEXTS

- Hegde, M. N., & Davis, D. (1999). *Clinical methods and practicum in speech-language pathology.* San Diego, CA: Singular Publishing Group. www.singpub.com.

Unique service delivery demands of schools, hospitals, and correctional facilities. Includes sections on general preclinic requirements, health and safety precautions, and assessment of individuals from diverse cultural and linguistic backgrounds.

- Goldberg, S.A. (1997). *Clinical skills for speech-language pathologists.* San Diego, CA: Singular Publishing Group. www.singpub.com.

An introduction to therapy, including technical foundational skills, complex skills, and qualities of master clinicians.

- Minifie, F. D. (1994). *Introduction to communication sciences and disorders.* San Diego, CA: Singular Publishing Group. www.singpub.com.

Refresher course on various concepts in communication disorders.

- Plante, E., & Beeson, P. M. (1999). *Communication and communication disorders: A clinical introduction.* Needham Heights, MA: Allyn & Bacon. www.abacon.com.

A lifespan perspective on disorders from infancy through geriatrics. Presents case studies to introduce and exemplify various communication disorders.

- Shames, G. H., Wiig, E. H., & Secord, W. H. (1998). *Human communication disorders: An introduction.* Needham Heights, MA: Allyn & Bacon. www.abacon.com.

Underlying nature of communication problems. Presents current theory, as well as procedures of clinical therapy.

- Van Riper, C., & Erickson, R. L. (1996). *Speech correction: An introduction to speech pathology and audiology*. Needham Heights, MA: Allyn & Bacon. www.abacon.com.

Nature, causes, and treatment of the major speech, language and hearing disorders including normal language development and professional issues.

- Klein, H. B., & Moses N. (1999). *Intervention planning for adults with communication problems: A guide for clinical practicum and professional practice*. Needham Heights, MA: Allyn & Bacon. www.abacon.com.

Problem-solving, decision-making processes in the context of selected areas of adult intervention.

- Klein, H. B., & Moses, N. (1999). *Intervention planning for children with communication disorders: A guide for clinical practicum and professional practice.* Needham Heights, MA: Allyn & Bacon. www.abacon.com.

Decision-making processes involved in clinical intervention planning across categories of children's communication disorders.

EVALUATION

- Shipley, K. G., & McAfee, J. G. (1998). *Assessment in speech-language pathology: A resource manual.* San Diego, CA: Singular Publishing Group. www.singpub.com.

Comprehensive presentation of speech-language pathology assessment methods and procedures.

- Hegde, M. N. (1997). *Pocketguide to assessment in speech-language pathology*. San Diego, CA: Singular Publishing Group. www.singpub.com.

Assessment procedures for all major communicative disorders.

- Haynes, W. O., & Pindzola, R. H. (1998). *Diagnosis and evaluation in speech pathology.* Needham Heights, MA: Allyn & Bacon. www.abacon.com.

Practical case approach to diagnosing and evaluating speech and language disorders. Includes both standardized and nonstandardized approaches.

TREATMENT

- Hegde, M. N. (1996). *Pocketguide to treatment in speech-language pathology*. San Diego, CA: Singular Publishing Group. www.singpub.com.

Treatment procedures relevant for aphasia, apraxia, articulation and phonological disorders, augmentative communication, and cleft palate.

- Hegde, M. N. (1998). *Treatment procedures in communicative disorders.* Austin, TX: Proed. www.proedinc.com.

Topics related to providing effective treatment to individuals who have communicative disorders.

AUGMENTATIVE AND ALTERNATIVE COMMUNICATION

- Glennen, S. L., & DeCoste, D. C. (1997). *Handbook of augmentative and alternative communication.* San Diego, CA: Singular Publishing Group. www.singpub.com.

Overview of augmentative and alternative communication including symbol systems and vocabulary selection strategies, motor access and visual considerations, funding, and legal issues.

- Lloyd, L. L., Fuller, D. R., & Arvidson, H. H. (1998). *Augmentative and alternative communication: A handbook of principles and practices.* Needham Heights, MA: Allyn & Bacon. www.abacon.com.

History and growth of the field, including development of assessment and intervention procedures, symbol sets and systems, access options, low- and high-tech communication aids, and current legal and ethical issues.

DYSPHAGIA

- Leonard, R., & Kendall, K. (1997). *Dysphagia assessment and treatment planning: A team approach.* San Diego, CA: Singular Publishing Group. www.singpub.com.

Review of major strategies for evaluation such as bedside, clinical, radiographic, and endoscopic evaluation in neurogenic, pediatric, and other populations of dysphagic patients.

- Logemann, J. A. (1998). *Evaluation and treatment of swallowing disorders.* Austin, TX: Pro-Ed. www.proedinc.com.

In-depth, cohesive approach to the evaluation and treatment of swallowing disorders from anatomy and physiology through assessment, treatment, and application to special populations.

LANGUAGE DEVELOPMENT AND DISORDERS

- Naremore, R., & Hopper, R. (1996). *Children learning language: A practical introduction to communication development.* San Diego, CA: Singular Publishing Group. www.singpub.com.

Overview of the language system including development of the sound system, meaning, syntax, pragmatics, and language diversity.

- Bernstein, D. K., & Tiegerman-Farber, E. (1997)). *Language and communication disorders in children.* Needham Heights, MA: Allyn & Bacon. www.abacon.com.

Focus on the ways children learn language and the ways to help children who do not. Presents theories of child development, speech and hearing science, and language development and disorders.

ARTICULATION AND PHONOLOGICAL DISORDERS

- Bernthal, J. E., & Bankson, N. W. (1998). *Articulation and phonological disorders.* Needham Heights, MA: Allyn & Bacon. www.abacon.com.

Eclectic perspective on the nature, assessment, and treatment of phonological disorders.

- Elbert, M., & Gierut, J. (1986). *Handbook of clinical phonology: Approaches to assessment and treatment.* Austin, TX: Pro-Ed. www.proedinc.com.

Survey of the clinical process from assessment to intervention and generalization.

NEUROGENIC DISORDERS

- Ferrand, C. T., & Bloom, R. L. (1997). *Introduction to organic and neurogenic disorders of communication: Current scope of practice.* Needham Heights, MA: Allyn & Bacon. www.abacon.com.

Current theories in the context of clinical practice. Presents a medical approach to communication disorders with emphasis on educational, social, and cultural factors.

- Hegde, M. N. (1998). *Coursebook on aphasia and other neurogenic language disorders.* San Diego, CA: Singular Publishing Group. www.singpub.com.

Includes chapters on dementia, traumatic brain injury, and right hemisphere syndromes. Presents integrated information on ethnocultural factors in assessment and treatment.

- Rosenbek, J. C., LaPointe, L. L., & Wertz, R. T. (1989). *Aphasia, a clinical approach.* Austin, TX: Proed. www.proedinc.com.

Selected treatment methods and applications for greatest efficacy.

- Helm-Estabrooks, N., & Albert, M. (1991). *Manual of aphasia therapy.* Austin, TX: Pro-Ed. www.proedinc.com.

Neuroanatomical and neuropathologic bases and differential diagnosis of aphasia.

- Beukelman, D. R., & Yorkston, K. M. (1991). *Communication disorders following traumatic brain injury: Management of cognitive, language and motor impairments.* Austin, TX: Pro Ed. www.proedinc.com.

Cognitive, neuromotor, and language effects on communication and swallowing following traumatic brain injury, including clinical procedures for assessment and management.

PROFESSIONAL ISSUES

- Pannbacker, M., Middleton, G. F., & Vekovius, G. T. (1995). *Ethical practices in speech-language pathology and audiology.* San Diego, CA: Singular Publishing Group. www.singpub.com.

Overview of ethics and values with academic and clinical case studies.

- Lubinski, R., & Frattali, C. (1994). *Professional issues in speech-language pathology and audiology* (2nd ed.). San Diego, CA: Singular Thomson Learning. www.singpub.com.

Overview of the professions including professional issues in health care and school settings and quality of care issues.

- Silverman, F. (1999). *Professional issues in speech-language pathology and audiology.* Needham Heights, MA: Allyn & Bacon. www.abacon.com.

Key professional issues currently under discussion in the field.

FLUENCY

- Bloodstein, O. (1996). *A handbook on stuttering.* San Diego, CA: Singular Publishing Group. www.singpub.com.

Theories of stuttering including early stuttering and normal disfluency and treatment procedures.

- Curlee, R. F., & Siegel, G. M. (1997). *The nature and treatment of stuttering: New directions.* Needham Heights, MA: Allyn & Bacon. www.abacon.com.

Assessment and management procedures currently employed with children and adults who stutter.

- Shapiro, D. A. (1999). *Stuttering intervention.* Austin, TX: Pro-Ed. www.proedinc.com.

Specific clinical procedures from an interdisciplinary perspective including multicultural issues.

VOICE

- Glenn, E. C., Glenn, P. J., & Forman, S. (1998). *Your voice and articulation.* Needham Heights, MA: Allyn & Bacon. www.abacon.com.

Anatomy and physiology of the human voice including sounds of American English, vocal elements such as pitch, volume, rate, and vocal color.

- Case, J. L. (1996). *Clinical management of voice disorders.* Austin, TX: Pro-Ed. www.proedinc.com.

Evaluation and treatment of the most commonly observed voice disorders in school and clinical settings. Covers basic anatomy, physiology, and phonation theory, evaluation procedures, spectrography, electroglottography, endoscopy, and stroboscopy.

MULTICULTURAL ISSUES

- Battle, D. (1998). *Communication disorders in multicultural populations.* Newton, MA: Butterworth-Heinemann.

Discusses the nature of cultural diversity and implications for clinical practice including a survey of diagnosis and treatment of each disorder for specific major cultural groups.

- Coleman, T. (2000). *Clinical management of communication disorders in culturally diverse children.* Boston, MA: Allyn & Bacon. www.abacon.com.

Key concepts and terminology with culturally appropriate assessment and intervention practices for multicultural populations in general.

- Roseberry-McKibbin, C. (1995). *Multicultural students with special language needs: Practical strategies for assessment and intervention.* Oceanside, CA: Academic Communication Associates.

Overview of cultural and linguistic influences on clinical service for various multicultural populations. Assessment and intervention strategies are included.

AREAS OF EMPHASIS FOR STUDY

Many individuals presume that they should study their weakest areas or study most in the most difficult courses. This strategy is not recommended in preparation for the Praxis for two reasons. First, no more than 10 to 12 questions from any specific area of coursework will appear on the Praxis. Therefore it is possible to successfully take the examination even if you are weak in a specific area of coursework. Second, questions from courses which are sometimes most difficult—for example, Anatomy—are not presented for specific recall. Instead, a question may test your knowledge of anatomy in the context of a clinical example. Thus it would be prudent to study anatomy in the context of a disorder; for example, anatomy of voice disorders.

The following is a list of specific courses that are not examined directly. Hence they should not be emphasized for extensive study.

Anatomy and Physiology
Statistics
Neuroanatomy
Research Methodology
Psycholinguistics
Phonetics

There may be some areas of knowledge for which you have not had specific coursework. The list below contains areas that are definitely included and that are strongly recommended for emphasis as you review your coursework.

Multicultural Issues
Speech Science
Language Development
Ethics/Professional Issues
General Linguistics
Dysphagia

Broad areas of disorder categories are emphasized such as neurogenic disorders, language disabilities, and fluency disorders, rather than specific medical conditions. Therefore, less emphasis may be given to the following.

Cerebral Palsy
Cleft Palate
Autism
Mental Retardation

RECOMMENDED STUDY TIPS

- Be familiar with all the content areas of the examination and the number of questions per content area. You will obtain information about the Praxis and a booklet of practice questions from Educational Testing Service upon registration for the examination.
- GET ORGANIZED! Begin to study at least 2 or 3 months prior to the examination date. Plan a schedule of what areas you will study each week. Adopt a regular and realistic study routine. Set aside a number of hours per week for study. Discipline yourself to keep to your study routine. If you miss any study hours, make them up at another time.
- Keep a daily study log showing the dates, times, and subjects you study. This will help you to see your progress, pace yourself, and know what areas you still need to review. Keep notes on any areas you may wish to come back to before the exam.

- Study both graduate and undergraduate coursework. Know the number of questions per content area, but do not base study on this information. You may need to study some areas more than others, but determine how much time to devote to each area based on your estimation of the number of questions in the content areas for you and the amount of knowledge you have in each area.
- Review class notes, retake old examinations, and look at textbooks other than the ones used in your classes. Memorize important facts, but also seek to understand and integrate the material so that it will be thoroughly comprehended and retained. Put facts that you may wish to review just before the examination on index cards.
- If you are studying for your master's degree comprehensive examination, remember that the Praxis will cover material from undergraduate courses as well. In addition, the knowledge required for the Praxis may be more general in nature than that of the master's examination. Therefore you may need to alter your study strategies to meet the demands of each test.
- Know those areas of the examination for which you may not have had specific coursework: e.g., augmentative communication, speech science, multicultural issues, dysphagia. Become familiar with this material.
- Form study groups of at least two other people. Exchange notes with other students, especially those from other universities. Make your own difficult examinations within the study group and quiz each other. Discuss the answers.
- If you have been away from your master's degree study for an extended length of time, a review course may be advisable. If a review course is not an option, select any introductory text. Texts with accompanying study guides are most helpful. Even if you attend a review course an introductory text is advisable.
- Don't study to memorize facts, although some factual information is necessary. Instead, study to update your knowledge. Visualize how information can be used in a clinical setting.
- Don't put more emphasis on the subjects that were difficult for you. Rather, emphasize the areas of coursework you are lacking.

UNIT 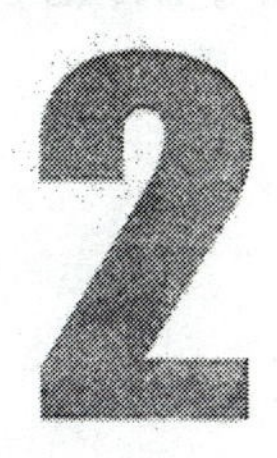

MISCONCEPTIONS AND FACTS

Gathering knowledge and information about the nature of the Praxis is an effective study strategy. Since standardized tests such as the Praxis are unlike the classroom examinations with which you are most familiar, it is of utmost importance to have a thorough understanding of the nature of standardized tests in order to maximize your performance.

Traditionally, there have been many rumors and misconceptions resulting from a lack of knowledge and understanding of standardized tests. The greatest danger of these misconceptions is that they contribute to test anxiety, which has the possibility of diminishing performance. The effect of misconceptions can be so strong that, even in the face of evidence to the contrary, some examinees cling persistently to the falsehoods, creating unnecessary and often deleterious coping mechanisms.

A list of common misconceptions about the Praxis is presented below, followed by a list of facts. The list of misconceptions probably could be expanded indefinitely. The best advice is to read all information about the test and mistrust any accounts that are inconsistent with the written information.

MISCONCEPTIONS

- **The best time to take the Praxis is after the Clinical Fellowship Year.**

The most optimal time to take the Praxis is near the end of your master's program. Students in training typically receive higher scores than nonstudents.

- **You cannot study for the Praxis.**

Many questions on the Praxis require recall of specific subject matter. Most questions require use of your specific knowledge for solving clinical problems.

- **You cannot write in the examination booklet.**

The test makers suggest that you mark questions in the examination booklet for reference.

- **You can only take the Praxis three times.**

Neither ASHA nor ETS restricts the number of times that the Praxis may be taken.

- **If you are not sure of an answer, leave it blank.**

Answer all questions, even if you take a wild guess.

- **You don't have to answer more than (some fraction) of the questions to pass.**

Strive to answer all questions to increase your performance. Don't leave any answers blank.

- **The examination always has an emphasis (e.g., dysphagia, audiology)**

A set number of questions is assigned to each content area. No area is disproportionally represented.

- **The examination is only on master's degree level study.**

The scope of the examination includes both undergraduate and master's study.

- **You should not indicate your race.**

Supplying this information is optional, but will not affect the scoring of your examination.

- **ETS knows who you are, and they will not let you pass the examination if they don't want to.**

Most standardized tests are scored and reported by machine.

- **You cannot take the examination if you don't have a master's degree.**

The Praxis may be taken by those without a master's degree.

- **You must report your score to ASHA every time you take the examination.**

At the time of the examination, you may select to have scores sent to you or to any institution you designate. Scores are sent only to the institutions you designate.

- **Every examination has a whole new set of questions.**

Some questions are repeated from previous examinations.

- **Some schools have the examination to pass out to their students before the test.**

The Praxis is security protected and is not available for early distribution.

- **If you don't pass the examination, you cannot get a job in the field.**

Not every job requires the examination.

FACTS

- There are 150 questions.
- You are given 2 hours to complete the examination.

- You have less than 1 minute per question.
- All questions are multiple choice.
- All questions have five answer choices.
- There is no penalty for guessing.
- You will need a score of 600 to pass the examination.
- You can pass by correctly answering 60–65% of the questions.
- The examination covers both undergraduate and graduate study.
- Most questions on the Praxis are not recall questions (e.g., you may be given an example or a clinical scenario and asked to make judgments, identify, classify, or interpret information).
- The Praxis may contain spectrograms, tympanograms, and audiograms that you will be required to analyze and interpret.
- Many questions on the Praxis will require you to make clinical judgments or use common sense.
- Optimal performance of the Praxis requires knowledge of content information, critical judgment, quick timing, and effective guessing.
- Negative stem questions (questions containing the words NOT, LEAST, EXCEPT) as well as Roman Numeral questions are included on the examination.

A topical outline of the Praxis is presented below as extracted from the Educational Testing Service, 1995. This outline gives the major content areas for the examination, as well as information to be probed within each area. The Praxis contains two broad categories, Evaluation and Remediation. Within these categories, however, a wide variety of information is probed, including each disorder, its nature, assessment, and remediation, as well as administrative issues pertaining to ethical practice and decision making regarding client disposition. Examinees should be familiar with the examination outline as essential information about the nature of the Praxis.

Praxis in Speech-Language Pathology Test Content Specifications

I. Evaluation (29%; 43–44 questions)

A. Screening

1. Normal development of speech and language
   a. Preschool language
   b. Preschool fluency
2. Hearing screening of school-age children
3. Referral/Ethics (i.e., role of the speech-language pathologist in screening geriatric persons)
4. Procedures for speech-language screening
   a. Infants—precommunication skills
   b. School-age phonology

B. Pre-Evaluation Planning

1. Etiologic factors (e.g., congenital cleft palate, voice abuse)
2. Referral materials from other agencies (basic science, instrumentation, age group)
3. Idiosyncratic factors (communicative differences and dialects and school-age nonverbal augmentative communication)

C. Case History

1. Interviewing techniques and interpersonal skills
   a. Adult voice problems—habits and work environments
   b. Interviewing parents of a noncommunicative child or of a mentally retarded preschool child
2. Establishing clients' past and present status
   a. Normal development of speech and language (i.e., school-age articulation/phonology problems, cerebral palsy, aphasia)
   b. Normal processes (delayed, central nervous system [CNS] function)
3. Knowledge of disorders to be elicited during the interview process (delayed articulation, adult fluency, school-age language)

D. Selection and Administration of Evaluation Methods

1. Test construction principles (psychometrics) related to standardization, reliability, and validity
2. Test materials
   a. Factors involved in selecting tests
   b. Determining appropriateness of selected tests
   c. Impact of communicative differences/dialects on test selection and use
3. Instrumentation (purposes and uses of electronic instrumentation for diagnosing a specific problem)
4. Nonstandardized procedures (language samples, behavioral observations, selection of appropriate activities for an age group or a disorder)
5. Ethics (issues such as right to privacy, needed permissions, IDEA)
6. Staffing
   a. Determination of reliability of assessment results
   b. Determination of intra- and interjudge reliability

E. Interpretation of Evaluation Results

1. Identification of disorder: type and severity
   a. Differential or definitive diagnosis
   b. Disorders related to adults

(1) Dysarthria, apraxia of speech, aphasia

(2) Right hemisphere v. left hemisphere disorders

c. Disorders related to children

(1) Adolescent language disorders

(2) Childhood problems such as developmental disorders (autism, multiply handicapped, cluttering, stuttering)

2. Formulation of recommendations
   a. Preparation for making a recommendation
   b. Impact on life conditions
   c. Type of treatment recommended
   d. What service delivery model is appropriate

F. Transmission of Recommendations

1. Ethics
   a. Knowledge of ethics might necessitate referrals to colleagues
   b. Knowledge of standards of professional and ethical conduct relevant to the evaluation process
2. Interpersonal communication and counseling
   a. Knowledge of supportive and informational counseling techniques
   b. Knowledge of skills to obtain cooperation from clients, family, and significant others
   c. Knowledge of information needed by others (professionals, referral sources, clients, etc.)
   d. Advocating for a patient/client
3. Referral
   a. When to refer
   b. To whom to refer (audiologist, ENT specialist, etc.)
   c. Use of appropriate terminology
4. Report writing
   a. What should be included
   b. To whom reports should be sent
   c. Use of terminology appropriate to the intended audience
      (1) Reporting to agencies about adults
      (2) Reporting to schools about children

G. Postevaluation Process

1. Monitoring as an ongoing cyclic procedure
   a. For maturation
   b. To determine if a client seeks suggested additional help

2. Diagnostic therapy (continuing to determine clients' strengths and limitations over time while seeing them on a regular basis)
3. Follow-up (one-time re-evaluation after no intervening treatment)

II. Remediation (66%; 99–100 questions)

A. Planning Remediation

1. Establish remediation goals
   - a. Normal processes of human communication
     - (1) Anatomy and physiology of the speech and hearing mechanism
       - a. Preschool—resonance problems
       - b. Hearing mechanism—school age
     - (2) Neurology and neurophysiology
       - a. Adult language
       - b. Children
     - (3) Psycholinguistics; speech-language development
     - (4) Acoustics and voice—adult
     - (5) Cognitive development
   - b. Etiologic conditions
     - (1) Theories of predisposing, precipitating, and perpetuating factors
     - (2) Conditions that affect communication development
       - a. CNS disorders
       - b. Cleft palate
       - c. Apraxia
       - d. Autism
       - e. Mental retardation
       - f. Hearing loss
     - (3) Conditions that disrupt communication beyond stages of early development
       - a. Head trauma
       - b. Acquired hearing loss
       - c. Progressive disease
       - d. Laryngectomy
   - c. Associated factors such as educational, vocational, social, psychological, and communicative effects on treatment programs
   - d. Types of disorders
     - (1) Articulation/phonology
       - a. Normal hearing
       - b. Hearing impaired

- (2) Voice and resonance
- (3) Fluency
- (4) Child language
  - a. Verbal
  - b. Nonverbal
- (5) Adult language

2. Selection of methods and strategies
   - a. Methods
     - (1) Behavior modification
     - (2) Developmental
     - (3) Computer applications
     - (4) Augmentative
     - (5) Motor
     - (6) Linguistic
   - b. Related factors
     - (1) Cultural and socioeconomic factors
     - (2) Educational, vocational, social, psychological status
   - c. Service delivery models (i.e., individual, group, consultation, isolated, integrated, etc.)
3. Determining termination criteria based on prognosis, progress, and motivation

B. Communicating

1. Informing and counseling about treatment plan to families, clients, significant others, and agencies
   - a. Information dissemination of legislation, guidelines, regulations, and requirements related to service delivery
   - b. Affects of counseling/guidance on treatment program
2. Procedures for referral and follow-up

C. Implementation of Treatment

1. Implement treatment procedures as specified in long-term goals and short-term objectives
   - a. Treatment methods and strategies for the following types of disorders
     - (1) Articulation/phonology
       - a. developmental
       - b. organically based

- (2) Voice and resonance
  - a. functional
  - b. organic
- (3) Fluency
- (4) Child Development
  - a. content (semantics)
  - b. form (syntax)
  - c. use (pragmatics, semantics, discourse)
- (5) Adult language
  - a. aphasia
  - b. traumatic brain injury
  - c. progressive disorders
  - d. acquired hearing loss
- (6) Nonverbal disorders (i.e., total communication, augmentative)

b. Procedures related to treatment continuum

- (1) Acquisition stage
- (2) Generalization state
- (3) Termination criteria

2. Monitoring client progress
   - a. Data gathering
   - b. Data interpretation
   - c. Documentation of progress

III. Administration (5%; 7–8 questions)

A. Ensure Quality Client Care

B. Advocacy and Interdisciplinary Interaction

C. Identify Individuals at Risk

D. Ratio Between Clients and Practitioner

Reference

Educational Testing Service. (1995). *A guide to the NTE Speech-Language Pathology Specialty Area Test. Part two: Test content specifications* (pp. 9–10). Princeton, NJ: Author.

UNIT

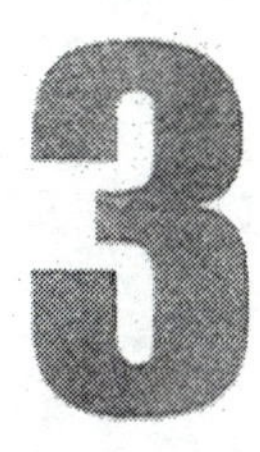

COGNITIVE ABILITIES

We have all observed how some people do well on examinations without ever seeming to study, while others study extensively without similar success. This phenomenon perhaps is due to the fact that certain examinations are constructed to measure "abilities," as well as knowledge. On these examinations the questions require the use of specific cognitive processes in order to demonstrate the required knowledge.

Examinations that test knowledge only are generally perceived by students to be easier than examinations that require cognitive abilities in addition to knowledge. One possible explanation of this is that studying can enhance one's knowledge, but no amount of studying can improve one's innate cognitive abilities. Similar to skillful piano playing, these abilities are developed only through practice and experience.

Cognitive abilities are those higher order thought processes that allow humans to use basic knowledge in a creative fashion. Note the difference between the following two questions as examples. The first requires basic knowledge, while the second requires cognitive ability.

Which of the following is a phonological feature of African-American English?

A. f/θ, initial position
B. f/θ, medial, final position
C. –/θ, final position
D. s/θ, final position
E. t/θ, medial, final position

Answer ________

Which of the following should NOT be considered an error for a 7-year-old boy who speaks African-American English?[1]

A. [pɛn] → [hɛn]
B. [pɛn] → [pĩ]
C. [pɛn] → [pɛ]
D. [pɛn] → [pɪn]
E. [pɛn] → [pʲɛ:n]

Answer ________

The first question requires knowledge of the phonological features of African-American English. The examinee must recognize the single correct answer among the other options. This type of question is known as a verbatim recall question. The answer is **B.**

Notice that the second question not only requires the examinee to know the phonological rules of African-American English, but the choices are presented within a word transcription from which the phonological rule must be extrapolated. The correct answer is **D.** This process of extrapolation is an important cognitive skill for the Praxis.

COGNITIVE SKILLS REQUIRED

The cognitive skills of the Praxis are based on Bloom's *Taxonomy of Educational Objectives: Cognitive Domain* (Bloom, 1957), which are as follows:

Comprehension

Comprehension entails grasping the meaning of material, converting ideas from one form to another, explaining or summarizing material and interpreting the meaning beyond data. Examples of comprehension include:

- Extracting the intended theme from written material
- Identifying and classifying the theme of written material
- Translating examples into concepts
- Identifying research examples as a type of design
- Identifying a type of hypothesis or statistical method from an example

Application

Application involves using abstractions in either general or concrete situations. Examples of application include:

- Making clinical judgments
- Making a prognosis for recovery
- Naming a clinical problem given its characteristics

Analysis

In analysis, the examinee breaks down material into its parts, identifies the parts, identifies the relationship among the parts, or identifies the way parts are organized. Examples of analysis include:

- Finding commonalties among symptoms then suggesting a treatment strategy
- Identifying the site of lesion by speech characteristics
- Identifying a muscle given the result of its action

Synthesis

Synthesis is the inverse of analysis. Synthesis involves putting concepts together to form a complete thought, production of a unique communication, production of a plan or proposed set of operations, or derivation of a set of abstract relations. Examples of synthesis include:

- Picking the best course of action in a clinical example
- Relating a kind of therapy to diagnosis and possible outcomes
- Interpreting and summarizing research results given in tabular or graphic form.

The cognitive abilities of Bloom's taxonomy are hierarchically arranged in terms of the complexity of the skills. This hierarchical order corresponds to the perceived difficulty of the questions on the Praxis. That is, the higher the cognitive ability required, the more perceived difficulty of the question. Figure 3–1 demonstrates Bloom's taxonomical hierarchy and the difficulty of Praxis Examination questions requiring each cognitive ability.

The easiest questions for examinees are those that require sheer recall of knowledge. Questions that require the cognitive abilities of comprehension, application, analysis, and synthesis become increasingly more difficult, as theses abilities

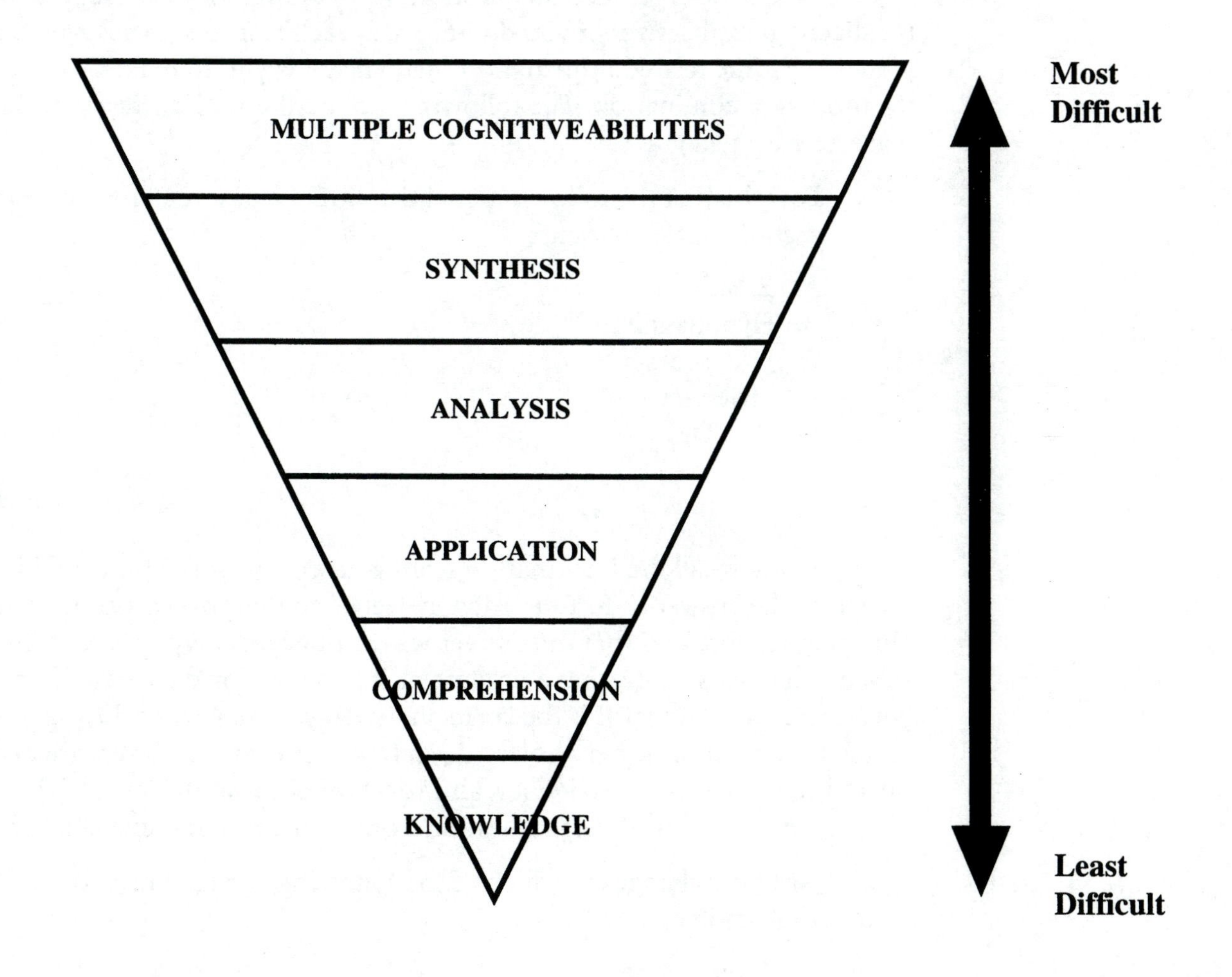

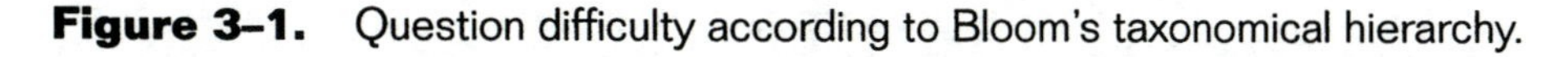
Figure 3–1. Question difficulty according to Bloom's taxonomical hierarchy.

require more complex higher order cognitive abilities in accordance with their level in the hierarchy. The most difficult questions are those that require multiple cognitive abilities which must be carried out in succession. Because errors of mental skill can occur at any level, correctly answering these questions demands a perfectly orchestrated process. Practice with each ability increases the necessary skill thus decreasing its difficulty.

RECALL QUESTIONS

Recall questions require knowledge of basic information from coursework. It is inevitable that questions of this type will appear on the Praxis. However, one should not expect the examination to be comprised largely of recall questions. Studying and memorizing facts will enable you to correctly answer these questions. But you can never recall all of the facts of the profession, and there is a great probability that only a few of the facts you remember will appear as questions. Therefore your rote memorization of facts should be complemented with other study methods.

One advantage of recall questions is that often they are easily answered by intelligent guessing. Even if you do not recall each fact specifically, you probably remember some related information that will allow you to make an educated guess by the process of elimination. The following is a recall question. Test your knowledge or make an educated guess.

For which of the following qualities would a nasometer provide the most accurate measurement?

A. Breathiness
B. Hyponasality
C. Hoarseness
D. Stridency
E. Vocal fry

Answer ________

If you recall the information from your coursework you would immediately recognize the answer as **B**. You probably feel good that this was an easy question. However, let's pretend that the answer was not immediately apparent. You could reason, merely by its name, that a nasometer is a measuring device for nasal emission. If you are not certain that B is the correct answer, you may work through the process of elimination with the other choices. A, C, D, and E would all be eliminated because breathiness, hoarseness, stridency, and vocal fry occur at the level of the vocal folds.

Answer the next recall question from your specific knowledge or by guessing.

Atrophic changes to which of the following is most likely to result in Huntington's chorea?

A. Frontal lobe
B. Hippocampus

C. Cranial nerves
D. Spiral ganglion
E. Caudate nucleus

Answer ________

If you recall this information, great. If you did not and you were correct after making a guess, good. If you were not correct after making a guess, note the flaws in your thinking, then refresh your knowledge. Of course, your answer should be **E**.

The following are typical questions for the Praxis requiring each cognitive ability.

COMPREHENSION

A 50-year-old teacher has been referred to a speech-language pathologist by her otolaryngologist. Results of indirect laryngoscopy reveal a slight bowing of the membranous portion of the vocal folds with vocal fold edema. The teacher reports that gradually for the past 6 weeks she has experienced increased hoarseness and lower pitch that advances throughout the day as she uses her voice. It is most likely that this patient has

A. contact ulcer
B. vocal nodule
C. laryngitis
D. vocal polyp
E. myasthenia laryngis

Answer ________

Questions that require comprehension are distinguished visibly by their length. A typical comprehension question is wordy and contains information for the examinee to read and interpret. In this question, the list of symptoms relate to a disorder known as myasthenia laryngis, so **E** is the correct answer. Note why the next question requires comprehension and provide your answer.

Which counseling technique is reflected in the following exchange between a client's parent and a speech-language pathologist?

Client: I don't know what to do. My son is stuttering severely and nothing seems to help. My husband just ignores the problem.

Clinician: I know exactly what you mean. My child stutters too. I just remind myself that dysfluency is sometimes a normal part of language development and he will probably grow out of it in time. Let's talk about how I can help your son.

A. Confrontation
B. Interpretation

C. Clarification
D. Paraphrasing
E. Sympathizing

Answer ________

This question requires translating an example into a concept, which is a skill of comprehension. The examinee must interpret and classify the theme of the dialogue. Or the examinee can survey the possible answer choices and match the choice that is most appropriate. The correct answer is **C** since the other choices do not characterize the clinician's statement.

Application

Application refers to the use of principles in general in a concrete situation. Examinees are often called on to apply diagnostic and treatment principles in clinical situations, as in the following question.

A 12-year-old girl with no history of palatal cleft demonstrates nasal escape and reduced intraoral pressure on fricatives and plosive sounds. Which of the following should be given top priority in clinical management?

A. Exercises to improve velopharyngeal valving
B. Referral to determine organic causation
C. Articulation therapy to increase intelligibility
D. Ear training to become aware of the problem
E. Mirror exercises to improve articulatory placement and reduce nasal escape

Answer ________

Here the examinee must make a clinical judgment by applying a known therapy principle of which approach should receive priority in management. Naturally, if physical structures can be repaired this should be done before the initiation of speech therapy. Therefore the answer is **B**. Apply your knowledge of principles to the next question.

The parents of a 4-year-old boy have expressed concerns about his dysfluent speech behaviors. The speech-language pathologist concludes that the child is exhibiting normal nonfluency. Which of the following most accurately supports this conclusion?

A. The child is too young to have developed dysfluent speech
B. The child displays no associated behaviors
C. The child's speech is 20% dysfluent
D. The child's speech is slow and hesitant
E. The child's speech is characterized primarily by whole word repetitions

Answer ________

Since the child is 4 years old, there is the probability that his speech will contain normal nonfluencies. Choice E represents the principle that is most appropriate to normal dysfluency.

ANALYSIS

Analytical ability relates to the capacity to think logically in a rule-constrained manner and to use common sense. Typical questions present a set of conditions describing a fictional situation that requires your logical and systematic reasoning in order to select the intended answer.

The Praxis may contain questions which call for analysis in several different forms. Bloom (1957) gives three forms of analysis: analysis of elements, analysis of relationships, and analysis of organizational principles. The following question is an example that requires both analysis of elements and analysis of relationships.

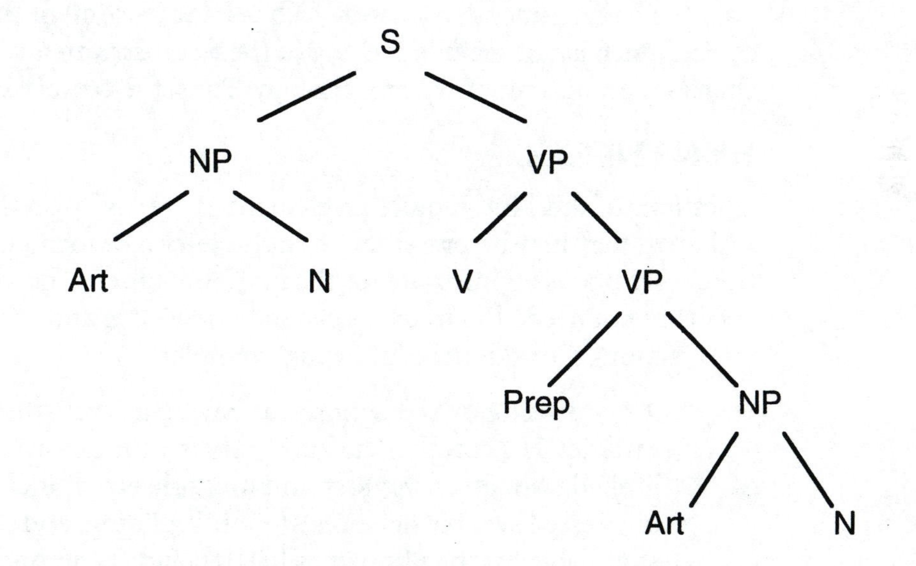

Which of the following sentences can be analyzed according to the tree diagram above?

A. An apple keeps the doctor away
B. The tree fell in the water
C. The man went there again yesterday
D. That is the one I like
E. I want you to be there

Answer ________

The examinee must analyze the characteristics of each semantic marker (element), as well as the sequence in which they are presented (relationships). First an article (*the*); a noun (*tree*); a verb (*fell*); a preposition (*into*); another article (*the*); and finally a noun (*water*). The correct answer, therefore, is **B.** Use you skill of analysis for the next question.

A clinician receives the diagnostic report for a child who has been referred for treatment of a language disorder. Results of three formal measures—the Bankson Language Test, the Carrow Elicited Language Inventory, and the Test for Examining Expressive Morphology—reveal an expressive language disability. Which of the following measures, if administered by the clinician, would add additional information regarding receptive morphology?[1]

A. Test of Language Development (TOLD)
B. Test for Auditory Comprehension of Language (TACL)
C. Boehm Test of Basic Concepts
D. Assessment of Children's Language Comprehension (ACLC)
E. Peabody Picture Vocabulary Test (PPVT)

Answer ________

The examinee must assess each test for its content then select the answer choice which is not included in any of the test instruments. Only one test among the choices examines receptive morphology. Thus, the correct answer is **C**.

SYNTHESIS

Questions of this kind require an element of creativity on the part of the examinee. Although they may be presented in multiple-choice format, the examinee must select the choice that is appropriate for the question. Often, knowledge of specific facts and recall are not needed as much as general knowledge and ability to propose a plan or set of actions. Consider the following example.

A 3-year-old boy is diagnosed as having a severe phonological and syntactic disorder. His comprehension ability is within normal limits; however, he has a limited phonetic inventory and multiple errors including final consonant and unstressed syllable deletion, stopping, gliding, and cluster simplification. He is stimulable for the phonemes [p], [t], and [n] in final position. Which of the following is the most appropriate treatment sequence?

I. Expand phonetic inventory by establishing fricatives [s] and [f]
II. Expand utterance length and use of grammatical morphemes
III. Establish production of final consonants in syllables
IV. Expand inventory of multisyllabic words

A. III, I, II, and IV
B. IV, I, III, and II
C. I, III, II, and IV
D. IV, III, I, and II
E. III, I, IV, and II

Answer ________

To arrive at the correct answer, the examinee must consider all the information about the child's language and devise a plan of action based on the most appropriate place to begin treatment. From the information presented, the child has both speech and language impairments. The phonological impairments are in need of the most immediate attention. Treatment should begin with sounds that are stimulable and proceed to more complex levels of phonological ability. Therefore, **E** is the most appropriate response. Using synthesis answer the following questions.

On a test of articulation, a 7-year-old child produces the following utterances

[fɑʊlɚ] for flower

[æmənəl] for animal

The phonological process exhibited by this child is

A. labialization
B. fronting
C. gliding
D. metathesis
E. epenthesis

Answer ________

In this question, examples are presented for the clinician to interpret and categorize. The correct answer is **D.**

MULTIPLE COGNITIVE ABILITIES

Some Praxis questions require the use of more than one cognitive ability. As the number and type of cognitive abilities required for a question increase in complexity, so does its level of difficulty. In fact, many Praxis questions are perceived as difficult not because they tap obscure or difficult subject matter, but because they require sophisticated reasoning or understanding. Consider the level of difficulty of the following two questions.

"No differences exist in the maximal phonatory duration of the vowel /a/ between subjects with ataxic dysarthria and matched subjects with a history of neurologic disease." The statement above is an example of[2]

A. an independent variable
B. a dependent variable
C. a null hypothesis
D. a research hypothesis
E. a theory

Answer ________

Cognitive Abilities Needed
Knowledge
Comprehension

A hypothetical study of children with articulation disorders is being conducted to determine which of two treatment programs is more effective in remediating a particular pattern of articulatory substitution. Thirty children meeting a number of criteria for inclusion into the study have been selected. The inclusion criteria assure that the sample is reasonably homogeneous with respect to a large number of variables that might influence the outcome of treatment, such as severity, age, and prior treatment. Which of the following is the best approach to assigning the children to a treatment condition?[2]

A. Having a panel of physicians assign each child to the treatment condition that the panel feels will be most beneficial
B. Randomly assigning half of the children to each condition
C. Allowing the children to select the treatment they prefer
D. Assigning males to one treatment condition and females to the other
E. Giving each child a trial session using each approach and then assigning the child to the approach to which he or she responded most favorably

Answer ________

Cognitive Abilities Needed
Knowledge
Comprehension
Synthesis

The answer to the first question is C. For the second question, the correct answer is B. Identify the cognitive abilities needed, then answer the following.

Research with language disordered children has demonstrated that their proficiency with grammatical morphemes is typically below that which would be predicted on the basis of utterance length. This suggests that[3]

A. The rules which are typically used for determining utterance length are inappropriate for use with language disordered children
B. Mean length of utterance is a better index of phrase structure complexity than of morphological knowledge
C. Language disordered children learn grammatical morphology more slowly than do normal children
D. Grammatical morphology is a relatively unimportant aspect of linguistic competence
E. Language disordered children acquire language in patterns of development which are different than those seen in normal children

Cognitive abilities needed ________

____

Answer ________

This question requires two cognitive abilities: extrapolation and synthesis. The synthesis ability involved in this question is related to derivation of a set of abstract relations. Much like the previous question involving extrapolation, the above question presents information or data from which the examinee must draw a conclusion. In addition, the examinee must use synthesis to discern the relationship between low proficiency with grammatical morphemes and utterance length. The question suggests that utterance length has a predictive relationship with proficiency with grammatical morphemes and that language disordered children have a slower rate of development of morphemes than utterance length. Thus, the only answer choice which contains a conclusion which is consistent with this reasoning is E.

Reference

Bloom, B. (1957). *Taxonomy of education objectives: Cognitive domain.* New York, NY: David McKay.

Sources

1. Educational Testing Service. (1982). *NTE Programs Ticketron descriptive pool for the Core Battery and Specialty Area tests* (p. 130). Princeton, NJ: Author.
2. Ibid., p. 131.
3. Johnston, J. (1982). The language disordered child. In J. L. Northern (Ed.), *Review manual for speech, language and hearing* (p. 287). Philadelphia, PA: W. B. Saunders.

UNIT

REASONING SKILLS

Standardized tests generally require the use of different operations than those that are usually sufficient for classroom examinations. In the classroom, many instructors write examinations to ensure that students have absorbed the needed information. Most classroom examinations are composed of "verbatim recall" questions such as the example below.

Prominent shoulder movement is indicative of[1]
A. thoracic breathing
B. abdominal breathing
C. clavicular breathing
D. pulmonary distress
E. hyperventilation

Answer ________

The above question calls for the student to use his or her knowledge of the subject matter to select the appropriate answer, which is C.

A common type of question found on the Praxis requires more than sheer knowledge. These questions may resemble verbatim recall questions, but actually much more than knowledge is needed for arriving at the correct choice. Consider the following question.

A clinician administers the Goldman-Fristoe Test of Articulation to a 5-year-old child. Upon presentation of the picture of a gun the child refuses to respond, saying "I can't say that. That's a bad word." In order to elicit the target sounds, the clinician could most reasonably

A. tell the child that it is all right to say the word
B. skip the word containing the sounds
C. insist that it is all right for the child to say the word
D. substitute another word containing the sounds
E. say the word and ask the child to repeat it

Answer ________

The above question calls for reasoning skills. The question is somewhat philosophical and perhaps even abstract. Indeed, any of the answer choices could be appropriate. The correct answer is D.

This unit discusses this kind of question and the reasoning skill needed to select the appropriate answer choice. Included are 12 reasoning skills required for the Praxis. This unit also discusses a typical type of question known as the negative stem question.

- Classification
- Fusion
- Comparison
- Cluing
- Predicting the Examiner
- Focusing
- Abstract Reasoning
- Recognizing Key words
- Critiquing
- Creativity
- Grouping
- Values

CLASSIFICATION

Questions that require classification are usually philosophical and abstract. The question itself may contain little or no information, while the answer choices contain the necessary facts. Classification questions require three distinct reasoning skills:

- Discriminating fine differences among answer choices
- Distinguishing quality and quantity aspects among answer choices
- Prioritizing and placing the answer choices in hierarchical order

Classification questions often contain words such as *best, least, primary, preferred, major* or *main*. The following is an example of a classification question.

The practice of speech-language pathology requires informed clinical judgments. Knowing which behaviors can change and whether individual clients can change is of primary importance for a clinician to[2]

A. implement appropriate clinical services
B. determine the best treatment schedule
C. know what referrals to make
D. offer precise prognostic statements
E. enable clients to overcome emotional reactions

Answer ________

This question requires the examinee to select the option that takes highest priority above all others by classification of the answer choices. The correct answer is **A**.

Note that in the foregoing philosophical, abstract question, the appropriate answer choice was also philosophical and abstract. The wrong choices were more concrete. Not all classification questions will present an abstract, philosophical choice.

However, you must utilize one of the three skills to arrive at the intended answer. With the knowledge you now possess about classification questions, answer the following.

In establishing management objectives for a 62-year-old woman who recently sustained a cerebrovascular accident, which of the following should receive the highest priority?[3]

A. The site of lesion
B. The rehabilitation framework
C. The presence of a right hemiplegia
D. Emotional lability of the client
E. An understanding of aphasia therapy

Answer ________

The rehabilitation framework relates to the client's overall life circumstances, including personal, social, educational, and recreational aspects. To arrive at the correct choice the examinee should classify the answers in hierarchical order to arrive at the correct choice, which is **B**.

FUSION

Fusion questions are the inverse of classification questions. Fusion questions require the examinee to find commonalties among the answer choices and select the answer choice that encompasses the others. Consistent with classification questions, fusion questions can also be philosophical and abstract, and the question stem may contain little information. However, fusion questions may not necessarily contain qualifiers or superlatives such as most or best. The following is an example.

To implement speech and language therapy the competent clinician must[3]

A. not use a method he or she has used before
B. develop rapport with the client
C. determine in the first session whether the client will respond to the method
D. have a complete understanding of the disorder
E. demonstrate a high level of technical and interpersonal skills

Answer ________

Answer choices A and C can be eliminated since they are untenable. To arrive at the correct answer, it must be recognized that E encompasses the other choices because in developing rapport and having a complete understanding of the disorder, a clinician would demonstrate a high level of technical and interpersonal skills. Use the reasoning skill of fusion to answer the next question.

A clinician conducts procedures to evaluate a school-age child with multiple articulatory errors. When analyzing the results of various measures, the most important observation for classifying the severity of the disorder is[4]

A. the total number of errors
B. the developmental lag in sound
C. stimulability of the error sound
D. the effect of the errors on intelligibility
E. the number of sound omissions

Answer ________

For the above question, all of the answer choices appear to be important. So the correct choice will be the one that encompasses all others. The correct choice is **D.**

COMPARISON

Similar to classification and fusion questions, comparison questions require specific reasoning operations performed directly on the answer choices. In many cases, the question appears to be the same as a verbatim recall question. However, selection of the correct answer choice requires more than sheer recognition of the answer. Comparison questions require the ability to discriminate differences and make evaluations of quality, degree, impact, or relevance. Of course, as the name signifies, these questions involve making comparisons. The comparisons are made among the answer choices as they relate to the information presented in the question. For example, consider the following comparison question.

Which of the following is most likely to result in hyponasal speech in an individual presenting a cleft palate and previously diagnosed velopharyngeal insufficiency?[4]

A. Secondary management that occludes the velopharyngeal port
B. A pharyngeal flap that is excessively narrow
C. Removal of adenoid tissue
D. Tonsillar atrophy
E. Development of Passavant's pad

Answer ________

This question requires the cognitive ability of application, as well as the reasoning skill of comparison plus application of the knowledge that excessive tissue within the velopharynx will inhibit nasal escape and result in hyponasality. The examinee must compare the qualities of each answer choice to select the one that most occludes the velopharynx. Thus A is the correct choice. Using the same type of reasoning, answer the following question.

Which is NOT a difference between single subject and group experimental designs?

A. Size of the subject sample
B. Need for control
C. Length of time needed to study each subject

D. Ease of implementation in a clinical setting
E. Concern for subject attrition

Answer ________

Using the skill of comparison, each answer choice can be tested against the others and ruled out or ruled in turn. Working through this process it becomes apparent that the correct choice is **B.**

CLUING

Cluing, or recognizing clues within the question, is a reasoning skill that is necessary not only for the Praxis, but for all tests. Often there are clues within a question which lead to the appropriate answer selection. Cluing involves the following abilities:

- Extracting relevant information from the question
- Recognizing key words or phrases
- Recognizing the appropriate answer among the choices

Clues may be intentional or unintentional. Examinees can develop a skill for recognizing clues within questions. This skill is developed through attention to detail and a conscious effort to find a clue within every question. Cluing is a skill that is particularly important for educated guessing, as well as for changing answers when you recheck the test. The following question contains an obvious clue that is perhaps intentional.

Examination of a 6-year-old boy reveals deficits in many areas in addition to articulatory skills. The most useful information for planning articulation remediation is gained from examining the client's[5]

A. physical status
B. related skills
C. environment
D. articulatory behavior
E. mental status

Answer ________

The clue in this question is "articulatory." Thus, the obvious answer is **D** in which the answer contains the same wording. A hasty examinee might overlook this clue, but simple reasoning would reveal that D is the only choice that is reasonable. The following question is a dead giveaway. First identify the clue, then answer the question.

Culturally sensitive and relevant procedures of speech and language assessment

A. Have been shown to have no impact on performance of culturally diverse clients
B. Demonstrate that performance of culturally diverse clients is consistent with norms

C. Are virtually impossible to develop and administer
D. Amplify the consistently poor performance of culturally diverse clients
E. Discriminate unfairly in favor of culturally diverse clients

Answer ________

The examinee should immediately focus on the terms "culturally sensitive" and "relevant." Naturally, the correct choice is **B**.

PREDICTING THE EXAMINER

Predicting the examiner is a practice with which students are quite familiar. In the classroom, students learn to recognize the instructor's style and what the instructor emphasizes or thinks is important. Either consciously or unconsciously, students learn to expect what will be presented on an examination.

One important distinction between the Praxis and classroom examinations is that the examinee is unfamiliar with the writers of the test. One should not assume that the emphasis or camp of thought presented in his or her training institution applies universally, or that the same textbooks for courses are used throughout the nation.

Predicting the examiner involves (1) selecting the universal or most socially acceptable response and (2) selecting the textbook response. Predicting the examiner is an important skill for individuals who are practicing professionals and who have been away from academic study for a prolonged time period. Often professionals develop their own personal slant, approach, or belief. It is necessary to recognize these and lay them aside for the Praxis. The following is an example of a question that requires the skill of predicting the examiner.

At present, no single theory explains the cause of stuttering because[6]

A. there has been no real attention paid to causation theory in recent years
B. well controlled clinical studies have taken precedence over basic research
C. the population of people who stutter is heterogeneous with considerable variability
D. stuttering is not sufficiently prevalent to be adequately studied
E. recent research has focused on treatment of the disorder

Answer ________

If you chose B or E, you did not predict the examiner, although your reasoning may be sound. You should immediately recognize choices A and D as most inappropriate since they would never be found in any professional textbook. Thus, your answer, and the correct choice, is **C**. Using the same logic, answer the following.

Children with language disabilities frequently evidence concomitant emotional and social disturbances. Which of the following is a true statement concerning clinical intervention?[7]

A. Since these problems can be expected to resolve with improvement in language skills, they need not be the focus of attention
B. Since these problems may influence the amount and quality of linguistic input to the child, they should be considered a legitimate focus of language intervention
C. The clinician must work around these problems since speech-language pathologists are not qualified to address them
D. Since these problems may disrupt language learning, intervention should not begin until the child achieves emotional health
E. Such problems are the consequence of hyperactivity and are best treated by medication

Answer ________

Several choices may reflect your opinion or experience. However, predicting the examiner requires the textbook or professional response, which is **B.**

FOCUSING

A common type of question found on the Praxis involves focusing. Focusing requires the examinee's keen awareness of what the question is really asking, or what the information within the question implies. Focusing questions may seem complicated at first glance. They may be wordy, narrative questions. Focusing questions may also present an example or a case scenario from which students must extrapolate information or draw implications. Thus, they are similar to questions that require the cognitive ability of comprehension. However, another component of focusing is the ability to summarize wordy questions into more concise statements. Consider the difference in the following two questions.

I. "No differences exist in the maximal phonatory duration of the vowel /a/ between subjects with ataxic dysarthria and matched subjects with no history of neurologic disease." This statement is an example of[8]

A. An independent variable
B. A dependent variable
C. A null hypothesis
D. A research hypothesis
E. A theory

Answer ________

II. "No differences exist between subject group A and subject group B." This statement is an example of

A. An independent variable
B. A dependent variable

C. A null hypothesis
D. A research hypothesis
E. A theory

Answer ________

Perhaps as a result of test anxiety, or other reason, some examinees may fail to translate Form I into its simpler counterpart, Form II. Note that the question is not concerned with ataxic dysarthria or phonatory duration of the vowel /a/. It is a research question, dealing with identifying a null hypothesis. Therefore, choice **C** is the correct answer.

Use focusing in both the question and the answer choices to answer the following question. A helpful strategy may be to make brief notes in the margin or underline important words and phrases.

A 46-year-old female patient is self-referred for a vocal examination. She reports that suddenly 6 weeks ago she began to notice a change in her vocal quality and that while speaking she feels that she is choking or strangling. Examination with a laryngeal mirror by her family physician revealed no abnormalities. However, the patient says that the condition is getting progressively worse. On the basis of these symptoms, the speech-language pathologist should suspect which of the following conditions?

A. Laryngeal carcinoma
B. Contact ulcers
C. Polyps
D. Muscle tension dysphonia
E. Spasmodic dysphonia

Answer ________

If you have grasped the concept of focusing, your translation should resemble the following.

A choking or strangling voice is symptomatic of

A. Laryngeal carcinoma
B. Contact ulcers
C. Polyps
D. Muscle tension dysphonia
E. Spasmodic dysphonia

Answer ________

In the first version an extensive description is given in order to establish the fact that the symptoms include a choking and strangling sensation. Of course, the symptoms relate to spasmodic dysphonia, which is choice **E**. Use your reasoning skills to answer the following question.

A 76-year-old man has recently been diagnosed with Parkinson's disease. His head displays a resting tremor that disappears during voluntary movement. He shows considerable difficulty initiating, continuing, and terminating movements required for speech and his sentences are marked by short bursts of rapid speech. His speaking is also characterized by monopitch, monoloudness, and reduced intensity. Which of the following most accurately characterizes the patient's condition?

A. Hypokinetic dysarthria
B. Flaccid dysarthria
C. Ataxic dysarthria
D. Spastic dysarthria
E. Hyperkinetic dysarthria

Answer ________

First, it is important that the patient presents with Parkinson's disease, which is associated with one type of dysarthria. The question could be mentally reworded as:

Parkinson's disease is associated with which type of dysarthria?

Of course, the correct choice is **A**.

ABSTRACT REASONING

A common type of question found on the Praxis requires the use of abstract reasoning. These questions usually present information or evidence from which the examinee must interpret and draw an appropriate conclusion. In speech-language pathology and audiology, abstract reasoning may require clinical judgment, application of diagnostic or therapy principles, and reading and interpreting charts, graphs, and audiograms. Abstract reasoning requires the following abilities:

- Discerning the implications of statements or conditions
- Making generalizations to novel conditions
- Applying existing formulas or rules to novel situations
- Understanding relationships among variables presented pictorially
- Deriving meaning from graphic displays

The following is an example of a question requiring abstract reasoning.

What would be the most likely effect on resonance of an enlarged adenoid pad?[9]

A. Cul-de-sac
B. Hypernasality
C. Hyponasality
D. Alternating hyponasality and hypernasality
E. No appreciable effect

Answer ________

For this question the examinee must discern the implication of an enlarged adenoid pad through use of reasoning and logic. The logic must be in perfect one-to-one correspondence and free from overgeneralization and conjecture. Logically, if there is enlargement of the adenoids there is increased tissue mass resulting in reduced nasal emission. Thus, the correct answer is **C**, which is the effect of increased tissue mass. Use abstract reasoning for the following question.

> Which of the following classes of speech sounds is especially vulnerable to deterioration in the articulation of a postlingually deafened person?[10]
>
> A. Stop consonants
> B. Front vowels
> C. Final consonants
> D. Diphthongs
> E. Initial consonants

Answer ________

Omission of final consonants is a common error in hearing impaired persons primarily due to reduced force requirements for final consonants and lack of coarticulation effects. Thus the correct choice is **C.**

RECOGNIZING KEY WORDS

A typical type of question found on the Praxis involves key words. Key words are superlatives, quantity/quality words, adjectives, or adverbs which are either crucial or merely stylistic elements within the question. Certain key words provide clues to selecting the correct answer. However, some key words may produce ambiguity within the question, and confusion or uncertainty within the examinee. A list of key words used on the Praxis is given below.

Key Words

Best Used in questions that call for value judgments
Signals that the answer choices can contain two or more plausible choices
Used when the answer choice has two components

Most Used with a qualifier (e.g., most reasonable, most accurate)
Almost always an important clue to select the answer
Not essential when used with "probably" and "likely"

Primary Quantity/quality words
Major Always important for selecting the correct answer
Least Signals the use of classification as a reasoning skill
Preferred
• **Main**

Either	Signals the use of classification or fusion reasoning skills
Not	
Might Be	
Other Expressions	
Primarily	Not key to selecting the correct answer
Typically	Use tends to be stylistic
Commonly	Used with hypothetical cases rather than direct/fact questions
Generally	Can be left out grammatically
Usually	Does not provide clues to correct answer
Probably	
Could Be	
Should	

Note that superlatives such as *most* and *best* and quantity/quality words including *primary, major, least, preferred,* and *main* are essential to the understanding of the question. In addition, words such as *either, not,* and *might be* provide a clue to the appropriate answer choice. Other key words, such as *generally, primarily,* can be confusing to the examinee if too much emphasis is placed on their function within the question. Consider the following questions that contain key words (shown in italics).

Functional articulation disorders are *typically* caused by[11]

A. poor discrimination ability
B. motor incoordination
C. unknown factors
D. phonological disability
E. psychological problems

Answer ________

Usually, insertion of the word *typically* in a statement implies that more than one element is applicable and the examinee must now select the major or main element. Indeed, *typically* literally means *usually*. In this question, the word *typically* is merely stylistic since none of the other choices can be categorized as functional except choice **C**, which is the only correct answer. Consider the next example of a key word that is stylistic.

Spastic dysarthria is typically characterized by

A. vocal nodules
B. unilateral vocal fold paralysis
C. overadduction of the vocal folds
D. asymmetrical closure of the vocal folds
E. lack of closure of the vocal folds

Answer ________

In both this question and the previous question the word *typically* can be eliminated since only one answer choice applies. Of course, the correct answer to the latter is **C**.

CRITIQUING

While it may be said that all examination questions involve critiquing, this reasoning ability deserves special mention. For all examinations, examinees must critique each answer choice in relation to the question, then select the most appropriate answer. The finer elements of critiquing involve the following processes.

- Determining the relevance of statements
- Determining and evaluating negative attributes
- Selecting the worst answer

Critiquing questions may require a relative amount of general knowledge in order to answer the question, as reflected in the following question.

Research has identified a sequential pattern of sensorimotor, cognitive, and semantic prerequisites for development of social interactions. In language instruction of severely disabled children, when a client acquires a prerequisite, the clinician could most reasonably[12]

A. assume that it is available for subsequent activities
B. assume that it generalizes to other response categories
C. use it to obtain attention for other purposes
D. use it as a prompt for subsequent responses
E. assume that it can be integrated with other responses

Answer ________

This question requires the examinee to use general knowledge about therapy procedures. In effect, selection of the answer becomes a process of elimination. The question may also be treated as a true/false question with the intended choice being the only true statement. Yet, what makes the above a critiquing question is the fact that the examinee must evaluate each answer choice for its truth or falsity, as well as its relevance. In this question, **D** is the correct choice. Using a true/false process, or elimination, answer the following.

Which of the following is the most accurate statement concerning the initial examination of an adult individual who stutters?[13]

A. The examination should be long enough and thorough enough to establish a differential diagnosis and plan of action
B. The examination must be at least 1 hour long
C. The examination should involve measures necessary to determine a statement of severity
D. The examination should continue until a procedure with which the patient can achieve fluency has been identified

F. The examination should involve a thorough interview with the patient's parent

Answer ________

Simply stated, there is only one true statement among the answer choices. Note, however, that the question requires a general knowledge about stuttering assessment. Most of the answer choices are not compatible with basic theory or practice. By critiquing each of the choices, we must arrive at the only correct answer, or **A.**

CREATIVITY

Praxis questions frequently present material in a different form than the way it was introduced in the classroom. Many questions on the Praxis present a clinical scenario in which the examinee's knowledge must be transformed into a plan of action. These questions call for creativity. Creativity involves:

- Generating novel thoughts or innovative ideas
- Generating a realistic situation from a theoretical notion
- Deriving means by which hypotheses may be tested

For the Praxis, creativity may be necessary for questions requiring location of the site of lesion from specific symptoms, or inversely, ascribing symptoms given the site of lesion. In addition, creativity questions may require the examinee to make a diagnosis or recommendation for therapy. Consider the following creativity question.

A speech-language pathologist examines a 6-year-old boy who was referred for therapy following reconstruction surgery for a cleft palate. The evaluation reveals presence of nasal emission only on /s/ and /z/, with all other pressure consonants produced orally. Which of the following is the most appropriate diagnosis?[14]

A. Occult submucous cleft palate
B. Stress velopharyngeal inadequacy
C. Phoneme-specific velopharyngeal inadequacy
D. Postoperative velopharyngeal inadequacy
E. Postadenoidectomy velopharyngeal inadequacy

Answer ________

Although the process of selecting the correct choice involves critiquing, even before reading the choices, the examinee may reason that remaining structural anomalies should affect other oral sounds, not specifically /s/ and /z/. Hence choice **C** is the most appropriate selection. Use creativity to answer the following question.

A clinician is most likely to obtain a naturalistic language sample in which of the following communicative settings?[15]

A. Observing the child reading in class
B. Observing the child in dialogue

C. Observing the child in direct interview
D. Observing the child's response to standardized language tests
E. Observing the child in a parent-child dyad

Answer ______

Of course, this question requires clinical judgment. The examinee must create a plan of action that yields the most naturalistic data. The correct answer is **B.**

GROUPING

Grouping is reasoning skill that has been proven as an effective test-taking strategy. Grouping is the inverse of the process of elimination. Answer choices are ruled *in* rather than ruled *out.* Thus, grouping involves finding commonalties among the choices that satisfy the specifications of the question.

Grouping questions are often presented in Roman Numeral format. However, grouping questions may also be presented in a format using terms such as *except*, *not*, and *only*. The correct choice for a grouping question can be a combination of items (e.g., I and IV only) or a single item choice which stands out from the other choices (e.g., A. apples, B. oranges, C. grapefruit, D. cabbage). In general, grouping questions are verbatim recall questions. The following are types of grouping questions that are typical for the Praxis.

The elements necessary for sound to be created are[16]

1. energy source
2. compression
3. transmitting medium
4. vibrator

A. I, II, and IV
B. I, III, and IV
C. I and III only
D. II and III only
E. All of the above

Answer ______

All of the following are parts of a neuron EXCEPT[17]

A. axon
B. soma
C. ganglion
D. dendrite
E. membrane

Answer ______

To answer the first question, the examinee must know that the three necessary elements for sound to be created are energy source, transmitting medium, and vibrator. The correct answer is **B**.

For the second question, the examinee must either rule out the single false choice, or rule in each choice individually. A proven strategy for attacking this type of question is to treat each choice as a true/false selection. The answer is the single false choice or C. Practice answering grouping questions with the following example.

Which of the following types of dysfluencies is associated with stuttering?[18]

I. Sound prolongations
II. Incomplete phrases
III. Syllable or sound repetitions
IV. Interjections
V. Broken words

A. II, III, and IV
B. II, III, and V
C. I, III, and V
D. III, IV, and V
E. I, IV, and V

Answer ________

The examinee should validate each of the Roman numeral choices as true or false. The Roman numeral choices that are true are designated by answer choice **C**.

VALUES

In speech-language pathology and audiology, examinees are frequently required to make clinical judgments wherein values are reflected in the questions. Typical values reflected in the Praxis are:

- Law abidance
- Fairness and equity
- Protection of client rights
- Professional decorum
- Team spirit
- Cooperation with other professionals
- Objectivity
- Respect for the scientific method of discovery
- ASHA position papers and Code of Ethics

It is extremely important that each examinee read the ASHA Code of Ethics. This knowledge is required for questions for administration. Also required is knowledge of third party payment regulations. At least five questions will relate to aspects of administration. These questions are very easy, but the knowledge is so specific that it is usually impossible to answer questions without the knowledge. The ASHA Code of

Ethics can be found in most current textbooks or in the *Asha* magazine annual reference issue. The following is a typical values question.

In dysphagia intervention, the primary concern of the speech-language pathologist is[19]

A. the patient's comfort
B. the patient's respiratory status
C. the family's wishes
D. the patient's nutritional status
E. the client's understanding of the task

Answer ______

Given the values of the profession, the examinee should immediately recognize D as the correct choice. The highest value of the profession is the life and quality of life of the client. Answer the following values question.

Which of the following is the most accurate statement regarding intervention procedures for language disabilities?[20]

A. Language intervention is not necessary in most cases of language delay
B. Language disordered children should be given precedence in a caseload over language delayed children
C. Therapeutic intervention is useless in cases that have a neurologic basis
D. The initial focus of therapy should be the development of language structures rather than social or cognitive skills
E. Early intervention for all children is essential

Answer ______

This question reflects a basic societal belief, as well as the law. The correct choice is **E.**

NEGATIVE STEM QUESTIONS

Negative stem questions contain the words, *not, least,* or *except.* These questions are sometimes difficult for examinees because they require a sudden cognitive shift. While most questions on the Praxis are stated in the affirmative and require the selection of the best or most appropriate answer choice, negative stem questions are the inverse. These questions require the selection of the exception, or the answer which is most *in*appropriate.

Usually, negative stem questions are grouped and presented with a specific set of instructions that signal the necessary cognitive shift. In addition, the negative words are capitalized. This organization may be extremely helpful especially to examinees who, in the midst of anxiety and timing demands, tend to overlook negative words or neglect to make the necessary cognitive shift. The best strategies for negative stem questions are the following.

- Underline or circle the negative word to reemphasize its meaning
- Select the answer choice that is incompatible with the others
- For NOT questions, treat each answer choice as a true/false proposition and select the one false choice

The following is a typical negative stem question.

Which part of the cerebral cortex would probably be LEAST involved in speech control?

A. Frontal lobe
B. Broca's area
C. Wernicke's area
D. Nucleus ambiguus
E. Sensorimotor cortex

Answer ________

To answer this question, it is important to recall that Broca's area is the part of the frontal lobe that is involved in speech control. The entire frontal lobe is less involved. Thus, the correct choice is **A.** Using similar skills answer the next question.

Which of the following is NOT a characteristic associated with apraxia of speech?[21]

A. Awareness of errors
B. Frustration
C. Left hemiplegia
D. Right facial weakness
E. Impairment of language

Answer ________

Since this is a NOT question, each of the answer choices should be designated as either true or false. The only false choice is **C.**

Sources

1. After Nation, J., & Aram, D. (1982). The diagnostic process. In J. L. Northern (Ed.), *Review manual for speech, language and hearing* (p. 138). Philadelphia, PA: W.B. Saunders.
2. Ibid.
3. Ibid., p. 139.
4. After Bankson, N., & Bernthal, J. (1982). Articulation assessment. In J. L. Northern (Ed.), *Review manual for speech, language and hearing* (p. 204). Philadelphia, PA: W.B. Saunders.
5. Educational Testing Service. (1982). *NTE programs Ticketron descriptive pool for the Core Battery and Specialty Area Tests* (p. 132). Princeton, NJ: Author.
6. Guyette, T., & Baumgartner, S. (1989). Stuttering in the adult. *Study guide for Handbook of Speech-Language Pathology* (p. 167). Philadelphia, PA: B.C. Decker.
7. After Johnston, J. (1982). The language disordered child. In J. L. Northern (Ed.), *Review manual for speech, language and hearing* (p. 286). Philadelphia, PA: W.B. Saunders.

8. Op. cit., Educational Testing Service (p. 131).
9. Peterson-Falzone, S. (1989). Speech disorders related to craniofacial structural defects: Part 2. In J. L. Northern (Ed.), *Study guide for Handbook of Speech-Language Pathology* (p. 120). Philadelphia, PA: B.C. Decker.
10. Calvert, D. (1982). Articulation and hearing impairment. In J. L. Northern (Ed.), *Review manual for speech, language and hearing* (p. 232). Philadelphia, PA: W.B. Saunders.
11. McReynolds, L., & Elbert, M. (1982). Articulation disorders of unknown etiology and their remediation. In J. L. Northern (Ed.), *Review manual for speech, language and hearing* (p. 212). Philadelphia, PA: W.B. Saunders.
12. After Turton, L. (1982). Communication and language instruction for severely handicapped children and youth. In J. L. Northern (Ed.), *Review manual for speech, language and hearing* (p. 241). Philadelphia, PA: W.B. Saunders.
13. After Guyette, T., & Baumgartner, S. (1989). Stuttering in the adult. In J. L. Northern (Ed.), *Study guide for Handbook of Speech-Language Pathology and Audiology* (p. 168). Philadelphia, PA: B.C. Decker.
14. Op. cit., Peterson-Falzone (p. 130).
15. Payne, K. (1989). Speech and language difference and disorders in multicultural populations. In J. L. Northern (Ed.), *Study guide for Handbook of Speech-Language Pathology and Audiology* (p. 269). Philadelphia,, PA: B.C. Decker.
16. Shoup, J., Lass, N., & Kuen, D. Acoustics of speech. In J. L. Northern (Ed.), *Study guide for Handbook of Speech-Language Pathology and Audiology* (p. 74). Philadelphia, PA: B.C. Decker.
17. Larson, C., & Pfingst, B. (1982). Neuroanatomic bases of hearing and speech. In J. L. Northern (Ed.), *Review manual for speech, language and hearing* (p. 10). Philadelphia, PA: W.B. Saunders.
18. After Freeman, F. (1982). Stuttering. In J. L. Northern (Ed.), *Review manual for speech, language and hearing* (p. 25). Philadelphia, PA: W.B. Saunders.
19. Robbins, J. (1989). Dysphagia and disorders of speech. In J. L. Northern (Ed.), *Study guide for Handbook of Speech-Language Pathology and Audiology* (p. 306). Philadelphia, PA: B.C. Decker.
20. Waryas, C., & Crowe, T. (1982). Language delay. In J. L. Northern (Ed.), *Review manual for speech, language and hearing* (p. 281). Philadelphia, PA: W.B. Saunders.
21. Kearns, K., & Simmons, N. (1989). Motor speech disorders: The dysarthrias and apraxia of speech. In J. L. Northern (Ed.), *Study guide for Handbook of Speech-Language Pathology and Audiology* (p. 152). Philadelphia, PA: B.C. Decker.

UNIT 5

READING COMPREHENSION

This unit is particularly important for individuals for whom English is a second language and reading proficiency in English is not high. This unit is also useful for individuals who do not perform well on timed, structured examinations.

Difficulty of examination questions depends, in part, on the reading level of the questions. Reading level is associated with the elaborateness of language, syntactical complexity, and amount of technical jargon in the questions and answer choices. Reading comprehension is a process distinct from the cognitive abilities and reasoning skills needed for successful test performance. Reading comprehension requires several complex mental processes that must be in simultaneous operation during reading. The following is a checklist of the mental processes required for reading comprehension.

- Concentration
- Absorption of meaning
- Knowledge of technical jargon
- Visualization or imagery
- Reflection
- Contemplation
- Evaluation (agreement/disagreement)
- Recall
- Association/identification
- Appreciation for metaphor, symbolism, style, sarcasm

Each of these mental processes is under the direct control of the reader. But, to improve reading comprehension, the examinee must be aware of the extent to which these processes are or are not in operation and practice the processes that are found to be diminished or lacking. Only practice can improve the mental processes required for reading comprehension.

The following exercise can be used to test your reading comprehension. Read the question and note your use of the mental processes in the checklist presented previously.

Below are two excerpts of opinions on the same issue by two eminent scholars in communication disorders.

I. The position statement suggests that the eradication of the dialectal utterance is inappropriate. Further, it suggests that the speech-language pathologist *may* also provide elective clinical services to nonstandard English speakers who do not present a disorder. According to the position statement, the role of the speech pathologist for these individuals is to provide the desired competence in standard English without jeopardizing the integrity of the individual's first dialect. I believe we do a significant disservice to social dialect speakers if we employ this approach—the do nothing strategy. Surely it is time for us to assume a more positive and vigorous stance than advocated in the position paper. (Adler, 1985)

II. According to the position statement, standard English is the language of specific institutions within society. Further, it is stated that individuals who seek assistance in learning standard English should have the option of receiving such services from a speech-language pathologist. *Imposing* standard English as a second dialect presumes that nonstandard English speakers cannot learn to code-switch without mandatory clinical intervention. What Adler proposes is not far removed from days past when dialect speakers were routinely enrolled in speech therapy to have their dialects "corrected." (Cole, 1985)

The two views of the scholars are best characterized by which of the following?

A. They disagree over whether speech pathologists should provide clinical intervention to dialect speakers
B. They disagree over whether dialect speakers should receive mandatory clinical intervention
C. They disagree over whether standard English should be the language taught to dialect speakers
D. They disagree over whether dialect speakers can learn standard English
E. They basically agree on the role of the speech pathologist in providing clinical intervention to dialect speakers

The answer to the above question is **B.**

Reading is a form of communication in which the reader is the receiver of a written message. In reading comprehension, it is the task of the reader to decipher the message as it was intended. Since the author of the written message is not present during the communication to clarify misunderstandings, it is expected that the conventions of writing have been adhered to so that the reader's comprehension of the message is facilitated. If the writer and reader have the same expectations for the written message, there is a greater likelihood that the message will be received as intended. Hence, reading comprehension is facilitated if the reader has some knowledge of the conventions of writing.

On the Praxis, short passages or clinical scenarios are presented for the examinee to interpret. It is important for the examinee to know that clinical scenarios present paragraphs that are usually developed around a central theme. Usually, a topic sentence, which is the first sentence, introduces the main theme of the paragraph. However, depending on the writer's style and purpose for communication, the topic sentence may be implied, or may even be stated last.

In paragraphs where the topic sentence is stated first, there are usually several successive sentences which bear a relationship to the topic sentence. These sentences provide supporting detail and further development of the main idea. The final sentence may be either a summary statement or a connecting statement for the next paragraph.

Paragraphs that have a topic sentence stated last are usually organized in such a manner as to build to a climax. Generally, the first sentence is the most minor in the sequence in which more and more information is presented.

There are two principles of organizational patterns for paragraphs: coordination and subordination. In coordinate paragraphs, all supporting sentences carry the same weight. In paragraphs organized by subordination, each successive sentence adds information or support to the previous sentence. Paragraphs may also be organized as a mixture of coordinate and subordinate styles.

For passages that contain more than one paragraph, the organization usually follows a pattern of progression from the general to the specific. Paragraphs may be arranged to produce an additive effect, in which more information relative to the topic is presented in each successive paragraph. When the reader is able to discern the general organization of the communication, general reading comprehension is enhanced.

With reference to the question presented previously in this unit, the two paragraphs are dissimilar enough in their organization that the meanings of each paragraph might be misconstrued by the reader. The first paragraph presents a mixed coordinate and subordinate sentence organization. Its topic sentence is clearly constructed, and as it is presented first, establishes the main theme of the paragraph. The word *further* suggests the second sentence will add supportive evidence for the previous idea. The third sentence carries the same weight as its predecessor in presenting more information. The penultimate sentence begins to conclude the paragraph by stating the author's opinion about the foregoing facts. The closing statement makes a bold, rhetorical statement indicating the author's opinion.

In the second paragraph, the topic is implied. But for the examinee it is reasonable to expect that both paragraphs relate to the same topic concerning ASHA's position statement. In addition, the second paragraph represents coordinate organization. This is perhaps the reason why its meaning may not be readily apparent to the reader. Each successive sentence carries the same weight and adds more information about the position statement. The author's opinion is stated through sarcasm in the final sentence.

EMPHASIS

An important distinction between reading and listening is the nonverbal cues available to the receiver of the message. Listening, of course, requires fewer mental processes than reading because vocal and visual cues may accompany the spoken message.

In the previous question, emphasis is provided for the reader in the form of italicized words within each paragraph, which provide clues to selecting the correct answer. In the first paragraph, the italicized word *may* suggests that the author is concerned with the fact that there is flexibility for the speech-language pathologist to provide clinical services to speakers of nonstandard English.

In the second paragraph, a similar concern is expressed by the author through the italicized word *imposing.* However, the word emphasized in the second paragraph carries a connotation of greater power than that emphasized in the first paragraph. This idea can be represented in the continuum below.

−	0	+
withholding clinical services	may provide clinical services (paragraph #1)	imposing clinical services (paragraph #2)

It is evident, therefore, that controversy exists between the authors about whether clinical services should be optional or mandatory. Without reading this emphasis, the reader might view the sentences containing the italicized words as merely adding information or clarity.

Not all paragraphs will provide clues to the author's emphasis. One must practice reading for emphasis until it becomes a natural process. An effective method for practicing reading with emphasis is to read each passage as if the reader is delivering a speech. Review each paragraph of the foregoing passage placing emphasis where necessary. Practice using the following exercise in reading comprehension.

> How is one to study an organ such as the brain? The major approach, of course, is to study its components and then try to learn how they function together. This is done primarily in animals rather than in man. The principles of neuronal function are remarkably similar in animals as far apart as the snail and man; most of what is known about the nerve impulse was learned in the squid. Even the major structures of the brain are so similar in, say, the cat and man that for most problems it seems to make little difference which brain one studies. Moreover, neurobiology is notable for the wide range of approaches and techniques that have been brought to bear on it, from physics and biochemistry to psychology and psychiatry. In no other branch of research is a broad approach so essential, and in recent years it has begun to be achieved. (Hubel, 1979)

The following statements are related to the information presented above. Based on the information given, select:

(A) if the statement is *supported* by the information given
(B) if the statement is *contradicted* by the information given
(C) if the statement is *neither supported nor contradicted* by the information given

_______ 1. Much can be understood about the human brain from animal studies

_______ 2. The theory of cerebral localization is unfounded

_______ 3. A snail's brain contains all the major structures found in the human brain

_______ 4. The science of neurobiology has an interdisciplinary basis

_______ 5. In terms of neuronal function, the human brain is more complex than other species

(Answers: 1. A, 2. C, 3. C, 4. A, 5. B)

If you missed any of the above questions, continued practice may be indicated to improve your reading comprehension.

READING SPEED

Not much can be said for improving your reading speed at this stage of your life. Throughout your many years of reading, you have probably reached a plateau where your speed is now optimal for comprehension of what you read. However, your reading speed can be diminished if (1) the material is above your reading level, (2) your concentration is lax, (3) the topic is boring to you, or (4) new and complex material is introduced to you for the first time. Reading speed can also be reduced if you are mentally tired, frustrated, or anxious.

The importance of getting a good night's rest before the examination cannot be overstated. With proper rest, if your mind becomes sluggish during the test, you will have the power to perk up. However, if you have not had sufficient rest, you will become more and more sluggish. With proper rest, you can also increase your reading speed for short periods of time, or for short passages, and still maintain your level of comprehension.

Timing is an important aspect of all standardized tests. It is not recommended that you speed-read the entire test in order to finish, but you can speed-read short questions where selection of the answer requires only recognition. Therefore you can save time to use with lengthy, complex, and difficult questions, which require more time for reading. The following recommendations are provided to aid in more efficient reading on the Praxis.

- Be mindful of the time limitation, but do not speed-read the test. Vary your reading speed for different questions.
- Increase your speed for short questions and for material that is familiar to you.
- Read at your usual speed for lengthy, complex questions, or questions that otherwise require more concentration.
- Glance at each question to decide whether the question can be read quickly, or if you should reduce your reading speed, depending on your reason for rereading.

CHUNKING

You were probably taught to read by a method that stressed reading every word individually. Initially, you were probably taught to recognize certain syllable and letter combinations in order to synthesize the whole word. As you became a more skillful reader, you were able to eliminate this strategy and recognize whole words by sight, and thus improve your reading skill and speed immensely. This strategy is known as chunking.

Chunking can be utilized to increase your reading speed for the Praxis. However, the chunking strategy is used for word combinations rather than syllable and letter combinations. You can learn to recognize certain word patterns and combinations on the Praxis that eliminate the need to read each word individually. The following are syntactical and word combinations which are typical for the Praxis. Become familiar with these phrases to increase your reading speed.

"Which of the following . . ."
"Which of the following is NOT"
"Which of the following is the LEAST"
"Which of the following is the most"
"Which of the following is the most appropriate . . ."
"Which of the following is the most likely . . ."
"Of the following, which"
". . . the most appropriate . . ."
". . . the most effective . . ."
". . . the most likely . . ."
"A speech-language pathologist . . ."
"The speech-language pathologist should"
"The speech-language pathologist should appropriately . . ."
"A clinician . . ."
"The next step"
"What is the primary . . ."
"What is the first . . ."
"What is the next . . ."
"The primary purpose"
". . . is generally"
". . . is primarily"
". . . is typically . . ."
". . . is the most important"
". . . is the best"
". . . is an example of . . ."
". . . is known as"
"The primary reason"
"It can be reasonably concluded that . . ."
"the initial"
"most accurately"

It is also important to become familiar with the structure and format of typical Praxis questions. As the instructions to the examination state, each question is presented in traditional question format or as an incomplete statement.

This organization has two implications for reading speed. In many cases, an examinee can learn to anticipate what must be done to arrive at the correct answer. For example, for traditional question format, the examinee may be able to mentally formulate a tentative answer. Holding this answer in mind, the mental process becomes one of matching the printed answer choice to the examinee's tentative answer. When the correct answer is recognized, the examinee need not spend excessive time evaluating the other choices.

For questions of the same word length that are presented as incomplete statements, the examinee must spend additional time evaluating each answer choice for its appropriateness. Thus, comparatively, incomplete sentences may require more time than questions in the traditional question format. The format can also be helpful for distinguishing questions that can be read quickly from those that will require greater time and concentration.

A useful strategy in some cases is to eyeball each question before you begin reading. If the answer choices are presented as one word or short phrases, the examinee may read each answer choice to obtain a preview or sense of the topic of the question. Psychologically, this preview strategy may also have the effect of providing cues to incomplete statement questions, and rapid recognition for matching the examinee's tentative answer for questions presented in typical question format. It is **NOT** recommended, however, that you take the time to read the complete answers for every question because this will only cost you valuable time in the long run. Remember, you should preview each question, but read the answer choices **ONLY** for answer choices that are comprised of one word and short phrases.

References

Adler, S. (1985). Comment on social dialects. *Asha, 27*(4), p. 46.

Cole, L. (1985). Response to Adler. *Asha, 27*(4), p. 47.

Hubel, D. (1974). *The Brain* (p. 4). New York, NY: W. H. Freeman.

UNIT 6

MENTAL PREPARATION

Effective test-taking requires a combination of cognitive, affective, and behavioral strategies. This section will discuss the affective qualities—that is, mental and psychological preparation for successful performance on the Praxis.

Throughout your educational career, you have probably been admonished to get plenty of sleep on the night before an examination. This advice is appropriate for the Praxis. The reason for it is simple. Since you will be in the examination room for more than 2 hours, it is likely that within this time you will become both mentally and physically fatigued. If you have had the proper amount of sleep prior to the examination, you can rely on your energy reserve to refresh yourself. If you have not had the proper rest, it is likely that you will have no energy reserve. Thus, you may become even more fatigued. This, of course, can have a deleterious effect on your performance. Test anxiety is a major contributor to mental fatigue. The proper amount of sleep will also help to combat test anxiety.

Believe it or not, diet is also an important component of mental and psychological preparation. Be certain to eat a healthy breakfast on the morning of the examination. But do not introduce new foods that your body is not used to processing. If you do not typically drink coffee, don't drink it on the day of the examination. Likewise, if you drink coffee, do so because your body is conditioned to receive it. But don't overextend either your food or coffee intake. Follow your daily routine as closely as possible with regard to wake-up time and the amount, timing and type of foods and beverages. That second cup of coffee "just to calm your nerves," combined with a high level of anxiety, may prove deleterious to your performance.

Vitamins, minerals, and herbs that improve concentration and mental alertness are recommended for intake beginning at least 30 days before the examination. This will allow your body to adjust and produce effects spontaneously. Taking new vitamins and pills, especially caffeine, on the day of the examination is not recommended. Nor should caffeine pills be consumed to help improve your study. Of course, you should not consume alcohol on the day before the examination.

Similarly, don't introduce new foods to your diet on the days prior to the examination. Be aware of how certain foods react with your body chemistry and avoid foods that may cause allergic reactions or bloating, constipation or discomfort. Do not alter your regular eating routines. If you must be on a weight loss diet, either begin your diet routine well before or after the examination. Naturally, you should not overeat before the examination.

Maintain your normal exercise routine. Tense or sore muscles can cause discomfort and distract from your concentration. Practice relaxation routines in the days prior to the examination. Remember that you will be sitting in one posture and constricting muscles that you may not have not exercised recently. Practice deep breathing exercises to relax chest and shoulder muscles and reoxygenate blood cells and brain neurons. Deep breathing can also serve to refocus your thoughts for better concentration. You can relax the muscles of your hand and fingers by flexing and releasing as many times as necessary.

Use the power of positive thinking to your benefit. In the same way that athletes claim the home field advantage and pep rallies boost morale, keep your associations positive and seek the cheerful support of others. Pump yourself up for the challenge. Banish negative thoughts, fear, dread, doubt, and anxiety. Devise your own affirmations and believe them wholeheartedly. If you are religious, know the power of prayer. Also seek the powerful prayers of others. Create a positive vision of the examination situation and environment. Finally, claim the victory by planning your own celebration activity and look forward to it.

TEST ANXIETY

Test anxiety is an unsettling, unpleasant, discomforting feeling one may experience in anticipation of or during an examination. Research has documented that some anxiety is good for test performance. Test performance improves as anxiety increases, but only up to a point. Some individuals respond to test anxiety with effective problem solving, and thus experience test anxiety as a positive force. This phenomenon can result in enhanced performance for all examinees if it is harnessed and controlled. Positive performance depends on knowledge of test-taking strategies, self confidence, whether previous experiences have been successful, and whether significant others feel confident about your performance.

With extremely high levels of anxiety, performance begins to decline. If there are factors operating to cause you to anticipate failure, test anxiety can become maladaptive and interfere with your performance.

Examinees may experience distress, confusion, fear, physical malaise, and worry. As a result they tend to respond with ineffective problem solving. Higher levels of test anxiety occur when:

- The situation is seen as difficult, challenging, or threatening.
- The individual is unsure of his or her ability to handle the task at hand.
- The individual expects and anticipates failure.

Because of such discomfort, persons who experience high test anxiety are often strongly motivated to find a means of escape and resort to various mechanisms of ego defense, such as withdrawal, projection, and rationalization.

Withdrawal can take many forms. For example, even though students are encouraged to take the Praxis during their last semester of graduate study, many do not. Also, if students do take the examination at the end of their graduate study and do not succeed, instead of taking the examination at the next administration, quite frequently they wait many months, if not years, to retake the Praxis. By then, their command of the knowledge required to succeed is much less than it would have been closer to the end of their graduate study.

Another frequently used defense mechanism is projection. Many repeat examinees are convinced that their past failure was deliberately planned by the "powers that be" who developed the test and set the passing score. As a result, they tend to believe the misconceptions about the Praxis which, in turn, perpetuates test anxiety.

TIPS TO COMBAT TEST ANXIETY

The following tips will help you reduce test anxiety.

- Become familiar with all information about the Praxis.
- Become familiar with information about test anxiety, its causes, and impact on test performance.
- Develop test-taking and problem-solving strategies.
- Learn to focus on and attend to the task at hand, apply appropriate test-taking and problem-solving strategies, and do not engage in negative self doubt.
- Reduce self-preoccupied worry.
- Release your worries before you enter the exam. Imagine that you are an athlete about to run an important race. Only concentration and drive will help you win, not worry and fear.
- Accept that some anxiety is normal and necessary for good performance.
- Practice physical and mental relaxation exercises before and during the exam as necessary.
- Take several deep breaths before starting, exhale slowly.
- Note any physiological reactions you may be experiencing such as nausea, sweaty palms, nervousness, rapid heartbeat, stomach tension, or neck tension. Relax the muscles of your body as you exhale slowly.
- Release all negative thoughts or preoccupations. Replace these with positive affirmations such as "I can do this," "I know the information on this test," and "I am prepared for this test." Repeat these affirmations as necessary.
- If the first question is too difficult, **do not panic**. Go to the second question, and so forth until you meet success.
- If others leave the examination before you are finished, don't take this as an indication that you are behind. Don't measure yourself by other people.
- Take reinforcement from the questions you can answer correctly. Forget about those you do not know. Don't bother to keep count of the questions you do not know.
- If time is called before you finish, use guessing strategies for all remaining questions.
- Keep your own time during the examination. Proctors do not always give 10 or 5 minute warnings.

UNIT 7

TEST-TAKING STRATEGY

Perhaps in the exercise in Unit 1 you noted that you perform better with fill-in, true/false, or matching questions rather than multiple choice questions. It is important to realize that the singular distinction among all these question types is format.

Matching and multiple choice questions both demand that you recognize the correct answer in a pool of different choices. These questions also allow you to eliminate some choices. True/False questions are similar in that you must make a single choice but only between two options. Fill-in questions require completion of a thought with immediate recall of the information.

If you are adept at any other type of question, you can use the same skills to improve your performance with multiple choice questions simply by changing your perception. In your mind a multiple choice question can easily become a fill-in, matching, or true/false question.

As you proceed through the examination, first formulate a tentative answer in your mind before you select the answer choice as you would for a Fill-in question. Next, search for your answer among the options, as you would for a Matching question. Remember that the answer may not be stated exactly as your formulation, but the idea should be similar. In many questions, this procedure will not be possible. Therefore, holding your original answer in mind, you can test each option against yours, as you would for a True/False question. You may even strike through the options as you eliminate each.

The following is a general test-taking strategy for improving your performance on the Praxis.

- Move at a quick yet comfortable pace through each question of the examination.
- Because guessing will increase your score, try to answer all questions on the examination. However, on your first reading, you should mark in the margin those questions you know nothing about with an X. Mark questions that you are unsure about with a question mark.
- If you think you know the answer to the question, but do not immediately find the answer among the choices, eliminate as many choices as possible. Use reasoning skills to select the most appropriate answer or if you can eliminate all but two answer choices, guess wisely between the two. If you know something about the question and can eliminate some choices, try to eliminate all but two and guess wisely.

- If you know the material, you should mark it with a question mark if:
  a. You have a memory block.
  b. The question takes more time than it should.
  c. You do not grasp the meaning.
  d. The question seems to be ambiguous.
  e. The meaning of a chart, graph, or audiogram is not apparent.
  f. You are certain of your answer, but your answer does not appear among the choices.
  g. There seems to be more than one plausible answer.
- If there is time remaining, attempt to answer the questions you marked with a question mark first. Do not attempt to redo those questions you marked with an X.
- If there is time still remaining, guess at the questions marked with an X, then check all answers, moving quickly to cover the entire examination. Be sure that each answer marked on the answer sheet corresponds to the appropriate question. Be sure to utilize all the time you are given. Do not leave the examination before time is called.
- Check your answer sheet every 15 to 20 questions to make sure that all of your answers are in the appropriate response bubble for each number.

Practice these strategies with the questions below.

1. Which of the following may best describe learning disaibilities?[1]

   A. A generic term that refers to a heterogeneous group of disorders
   B. A specific language problem with some concomitant dysfunction in reading
   C. A homogeneous group of children with primary problems in reading and writing
   D. A group of problems specific to children in the adolescent years
   E. A specific problem that is restricted to academic skills acquisition only

   Answer ________

2. Which of the following areas of linguistic knowledge seems to present the greatest difficulty for the language disordered child?[2]

   A. Phrase structure rules
   B. Lexical meaning
   C. Grammatical morphology
   D. Relational semantics
   E. Conversational rules

   Answer ________

3. What type of prosthetic device is often used in cases of inadequate velar movement?[3]

   A. Palatal lift
   B. Palatal plate
   C. Speech bulb
   D. Articulation development prosthesis
   E. Feeding obturator

Answer ________

4. A formal approach to the acquisition of language which is common in many schools for hearing impaired students stresses[4]

   A. mastery of silent reading
   B. the importance of observing children's language in informal settings
   C. more written than oral exercises during language training
   D. the importance of observing children at play as a medium for learning
   E. grammar principles through memorization

Answer ________

5. Which pathologic condition only occurs along the medial border of the posterior of the glottis?[5]

   A. Vocal nodules
   B. Vocal polyps
   C. Contact ulcer
   D. Myasthenia laryngis
   E. Chronic simple laryngitis

Answer ________

6. A variable with predictive power for prognosis in articulation learning is[6]

   A. stimulability
   B. oral and facial motor skills
   C. speech sound discrimination
   D. laterality
   E. kinesthetic sensitivity

Answer ________

7. Which of the following clinical hypotheses would lead to the most specific clinical design?[7]

   A. John is mentally retarded
   B. James' language disorder is related to a maturational delay
   C. Bob's semantic disorder interacts with his pragmatic and syntactic problems

D. Alex has a severe language formulation disorder at all language levels stemming from an emotional disturbance
E. Mrs. Smith has Broca's aphasia resulting from a cerebrovascular accident

Answer ________

8. Disturbances in execution of the motor speech act due to muscular incoordination or paresis are called[8]

A. diplalia
B. apraxia of speech
C. aphasia
D. dysarthria
E. anomia

Answer ________

9. All of the following appear to be viable explanations of developmental language disorders EXCEPT[9]

A. difficulties with attentional control
B. symbolic deficits
C. neurological dysfunction
D. restricted exposure to the physical environment
E. inadequate body image

Answer ________

10. All of the following are treatment approaches for young children beginning to stutter EXCEPT

A. negative reinforcement
B. eliminating physical stress
C. creating rewarding communicative situations
D. reducing sources of emotional distress
E. fluency enhancement

Answer ________

Answers

1. (A), 2. (C), 3. (A), 4. (E), 5. (C), 6. (A), 7. (E), 8. (D), 9. (E), 10. (A).

RECOMMENDED TEST-TAKING STRATEGIES

- Read *all* instructions and follow directions specifically as indicated. Don't reinterpret the directions.
- Strive to fit into the status quo. Don't think of yourself as an exception.
- Adopt an organized and systematic manner of thinking and reasoning.
- Minimize the effects of your personal experiences, beliefs or values. Rather, think of the common experiences of the profession.
- Actively combat any stress that you feel, particularly if it creates mental blocks or otherwise impedes your performance.
- Don't let your mind wander, particularly if you have negative thoughts. Return your focus to the task at hand.
- Use deductive reasoning in selecting your answers.
- Be aware of time. Conserve time.
- Place value on precision—there is only one right answer.
- Think hard, concentrate. Don't take a casual approach to the examination.
- Even if you have not studied as much as you would have liked, rely on your mental powers and the general knowledge you possess to give you confidence. Never let yourself feel defeated.
- Think of the examination as a means to an end, not as a barrier to your progress.
- Adopt the attitudes, values, and mental outlook of the test makers. Think of yourself not as a student whose ideas are either right or wrong, but as a knowledgeable, integrated professional whose ideas are accepted.
- Pay attention to detail. Expect that every detail counts.
- Apply universal diagnostic and therapy principles. Don't focus on exceptions.
- Look for underlying meanings and implications, but draw conclusions based only on a strict and logical interpretation of the evidence presented.
- Don't rely on your global, contextual memory from the classroom. Remember specific facts. Let your memory of specific facts serve as the basis for choosing or eliminating answers in the present context. In other words, *use* what you know. Recall and relate every small detail.
- Don't expect the test to present information the way it was presented in the classroom. Be prepared to apply information in a different context.
- Assume an active role in the examination, not a passive role. That is, put your mind to work to figure out the answer. Don't expect the answers to come to you.
- Once you have selected an answer, defend your choice using sound reasoning and the facts you know. If your choice is not defensible, choose another.

STRATEGIES NOT RECOMMENDED

Do Not:

- Start at the end of the examination and attempt to work backwards.
- Change your answers unless you are certain that your first choice is not correct.
- Answer questions based on your personal clinical experiences. The Praxis presents textbook clinical scenarios and requires basic textbook knowledge. Subordinate your personal experiences and utilize generic academic knowledge.
- Utilize strategies that you have not practiced or have not proved to be effective for you.
- Leave any questions blank.

Sources

1. Guilford, A. (1989). Language disorders in the adolescent. In J. L. Northern (Ed.), *Study guide for Handbook of Speech-Language Pathology and Audiology* (p. 196). Philadelphia, PA: B.C. Decker.
2. Johnson, J. (1989). Specific language disorders in the child. In J. L. Northern (Ed.), *Study guide for Handbook of Speech-Language Pathology and Audiology* (p. 285). Philadelphia, PA: B. C. Decker.
3. Peterson-Falzone, S. (1989). Speech disorders related to craniofacial structural defects: Part 2. In J. L. Northern (Ed.), *Study guide for Handbook of Speech-Language Pathology and Audiology* (p. 130). Philadelphia, PA: B.C. Decker.
4. Ferguson, D., Hicks, D., & Pfau, G. (1982). Education and hearing impairment. In J. L. Northern (Ed.), *Review manual for speech, language and hearing* (p. 414). Philadelphia, PA: W.B. Saunders.
5. Reed, C. (1989). Voice disorders in the adult. In J. L. Northern (Ed.), *Study guide for Handbook of Speech-Language Pathology and Audiology* (p. 223). Philadelphia, PA: B.C. Decker.
6. McReynholds, L., & Elbert, M. (1982). Articulation disorders of unknown etiology and their remediation. In J. L. Northern (Ed.), *Review manual for speech, language and hearing* (p. 212). Philadelphia, PA: W.B. Saunders.
7. Nation, J. (1982). Management of speech and language disorders. In J. L. Northern (Ed.), *Review manual for speech, language and hearing* (p. 145). Philadelphia, PA: W.B. Saunders.
8. McNeill, M. (1982). The nature of aphasia in adults. In J. L. Northern (Ed.), *Review manual for speech, language and hearing* (p. 263). Philadelphia, PA: W.B. Saunders.
9. After Johnson, J. (1989). The language disordered child. In J. L. Northern (Ed.), *Study guide for Handbook of Speech-Language Pathology and Audiology* (p. 256). Philadelphia, PA: B.C. Decker.

UNIT

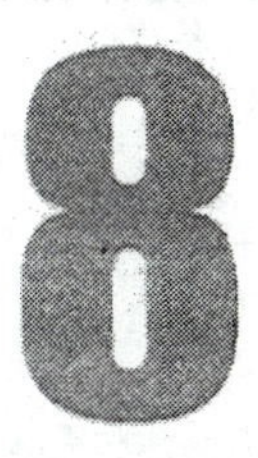

TIME UTILIZATION

For the Praxis, you will have 120 minutes to answer 150 questions. This means that you have less than one minute per question—48 seconds to be exact. Surprisingly, 48 seconds do not pass as quickly as you may think relative to examination taking. Some questions may take as little as 5 or 10 seconds to read, select an answer and record on the answer sheet. Other questions, of course, may take longer than 48 seconds.

Time utilization is directly related to your reading speed. It would be prudent to determine your reading speed before the examination, as well as the speed at which you answer examination questions. Use the following mini-examination as a diagnostic timing examination.

Time at Start: ________

1. In teaching semantics to a severely handicapped child, the words selected by the instructor should be[1]

   A. functional in the classroom and home
   B. functional and developmentally and environmentally appropriate
   C. primarily nouns that refer to objects and items in the environment
   D. phonetically similar to facilitate articulatory movement
   E. restricted to syllable and phonetic characteristics

Answer ________

2. Which of the following statements best describes congenitally hearing impaired children?[2]

   A. They are usually educated in regular school classes
   B. They have significant impairment of language
   C. They have normal articulation if they use acoustic amplification
   D. They are an extremely heterogeneous group
   E. They have a U-shaped audiogram

Answer ________

3. A 12-year-old girl shows academic difficulty related to language processing skills. If the child bears a normal range on a performance scale such as the Leiter, Columbia, or Raven, we must presume that[3]

   A. the child's intellectual development in nonverbal areas is age appropriate
   B. the child's intellectual potential is normal
   C. certain of the child's cognitive skills are age appropriate
   D. the child should be capable of age appropriate academic achievement in mathematics and logic as long as these subjects are taught nonverbally
   E. the child's rate of learning is age appropriate

Answer ________

4. Analysis of the articulation behavior obtained in assessment is completed for the purpose of[4]

   A. determining the cause of the problem
   B. selecting the target sound or sounds for treatment
   C. deciding the length of treatment
   D. determining the relevance of environmental events to the problem
   E. determining the presence of a language problem

Answer ________

5. Which of the following is not primary to clinical interpretation?[5]

   A. Integration and synthesis of constituent analysis information with clinical testing information
   B. Analyzing the clinical test information
   C. Utilization of knowledge of speech and language disorders apart from that collected from the client
   D. Determination of the accuracy of the clinical hypothesis
   E. Development of a diagnostic statement

Answer ________

6. Which of the following statements concerning ablative surgery of the face, mouth, and pharynx is true?[6]

   A. In most patients receiving this surgery, speech is rendered totally unintelligible
   B. Prosthetic devices may help to restore the normal size and shape of a resonance cavity
   C. Prosthetic devices cannot be used to reclose a resonance chamber

D. Unilateral nasal excisions will have no effect on nasal resonances as long as the contralateral nasal cavity is undisturbed
E. Ablative surgery of the pharynx is less deleterious for speech than ablative surgery of the oral cavity since fewer formants are affected

Answer ________

7. "Symptomatic" voice therapy emphasizes[7]

A. different techniques for functional and organic disorders
B. "restorative" techniques creating optimal conditions for the vocal folds to heal
C. techniques that facilitate the patient's best voice along the perceptual dimensions of loudness, pitch, and quality
D. the patient's "best voice" productions which are explored every clinical session and become the target model for him or her to watch
E. C and D above

Answer ________

8. Which of the following areas should be evaluated in the assessment of vocal dysfunction?[8]

I. Phonatory awareness
II. Articulatory accuracy
III. Resonance
IV. Respiratory function

A. I, II, and IV only
B. I, III, and IV only
C. I, II, and III only
D. II, III, and IV
E. All of the above

Answer ________

9. In evaluating speech and language, baselines are[9]

A. measures of behaviors in the absence of planned intervention
B. measures of generalizations of treatment disorders
C. measures of maintenance of treated behaviors
D. established before the assessment
E. less reliable than standardized tests

Answer ________

10. In the evaluation of stuttering, measures of rate[10]

    A. are somewhat complicated in that the rate at which words are communicated is not the same as the rate at which fluent speech is produced
    B. should include both words per minute and syllables per minute
    C. can be adequately estimated as low, normal, or fast
    D. need not be taken because therapy always involves reduced rate of speech anyway
    E. are not relevant to the quality of the patient's speech

Answer _______

11. Neurologic examination of a child revealed a left-sided weakness of the arms, legs, and lower half of the face. The lesion most likely was located[11]

    A. in the direct descending motor pathways (pyramidal tract) above the level of the decussation on the left
    B. in the direct descending motor pathways (pyramidal tract) above the level of the decussation on the right
    C. in the direct descending motor pathways (pyramidal tract) below the level of decussation on the right
    D. in the direct descending motor pathways (pyramidal trace) below the level of decussation on the left
    E. in the indirect (extrapyramidal tract) descending motor fibers

Answer _______

12. Based on observations of developing stuttering, we can say that if a child's stuttering persists[12]

    A. there is a strong likelihood of change in the characteristics of stuttering as the child matures
    B. associated or secondary characteristics will occur after puberty
    C. all stuttering characteristics will proceed on the same course of development
    D. we can predict the course of future development based on assessment of the child
    E. therapy can be planned according to a predicted course of development

Answer _______

13. All of the following are true with regard to articulation in dysarthric children EXCEPT[13]

    A. dyskinetic dysarthric children often present with more severe articulation problems than spastic dysarthric children

B. articulation error patterns noted in dysarthric children appear to persist into adulthood
C. research explicating articulation patterns in dysarthric children has been limited
D. vowel production is usually not impaired
E. hypernasality and nasal emission are common

Answer ________

14. Technically, the treatment in communicative disorders implemented by speech-language pathologists consists of[14]

A. a strict management of a relation between antecedents, responses, and their consequences
B. eliminating the neurophysiologic bases of given disorders
C. enhancing the communicative potential of individuals
D. removing barriers to social achievement
E. eliminating the original cause of disorders

Answer ________

15. Which of the following is a problem that might be investigated using correlational statistics?[15]

A. A speech pathologist measures the relationship between number of hours of therapy and recovery rate in aphasics
B. A developmental specialist notes the age at which nouns, pronouns, adjectives, and other parts of speech occur in the verbal output of a large group of children
C. An audiologist records the minimal differences between tones detectable by subjects with normal hearing
D. An experimenter compares language acquisition patterns in Black and White children
E. A researcher records the prevalence of speech and language disorders among various age groups

Answer ________

Time at Finish: ________ Total Minutes ________

Compute your timing as follows:

Total minutes ÷ (15) × (60) = Average seconds per question: ________

You should have completed this mini-examination in a maximum of nine minutes. Since you will need additional time at the end of the examination to recheck your work, it is advisable to not use the total time for answering questions. A good exam taker will have at least one half hour to recheck the examination. Thus, your speed should actually be 38 seconds per question. Note how your speed compares to this figure.

Answers

1. (B), 2. (D), 3. (C), 4. (B), 5. (B), 6. (B), 7. (B), 8. (B), 9. (A), 10. (A), 11. (B), 12. (A), 13. (D), 14. (A), 15. (A).

If you determine that you must increase your speed, it is imperative that you practice *before* the examination so that an increased speed will be comfortable to you. It is not recommended that you hasten your pace only for the examination. This unpracticed, uncomfortable speed during the examination may be deleterious in that it may promote test anxiety, as well as cause you to make mistakes in your haste.

The following recommendations are given for time utilization during the examination.

- Establish a comfortable speed for the first 15 minutes of the examination. After 15 minutes, check the number of questions completed. You should have completed at least 20 questions.
- If you have not reached 20 questions, hasten your speed for short or easy questions. Read long or difficult questions at your usual speed. It is important to hasten your speed early during the examination, rather than wait and increase speed during the final minutes. An early increase in speed will help you to reach the end of the examination so that you will have time to recheck to find any mistakes. Remember that guessing on questions you know nothing about saves valuable time.
- At the half hour mark, you should be nearing completion of 1/4 to 1/3 of the examination (38 to 50 questions). Of course, if you have surpassed this number, continue to work at a comfortable speed. If you have not reached 38 questions after one half hour, mentally diagnose your problem and take the necessary strategies to increase your speed. DO NOT PANIC. You may still pass the examination even if you do not reach some questions.
- After 1 hour you should have completed more than half the examination. Continue to monitor your time and progress.
- If you run short of time, do not stop to recheck the examination. Strive to complete as many questions as possible. There will be some easy questions toward the end of the examination.
- If you know that you will not complete the examination before time is called, work until the final minute. In the last minute, select any letter of your choice and mark all remaining answer bubbles with that same letter. Note: This strategy is not unethical, but is a useful guessing strategy that is guaranteed to increase your score.

STRATEGIES NOT RECOMMENDED

Do Not:

- Speed-read the examination.
- Spend excessive time on difficult questions.
- Daydream on other matters.
- Interrupt the examination to utilize the facilities.
- Be distracted by others.
- Stop to take a rest.
- Read the answer choices before reading the examination (this does not apply to one-word or short phrase answer choices for which you may take a quick glance).
- Leave the examination before time is called.
- Stop to recheck the examination if you have not completed all questions.
- On recheck, begin at question #1 and re-assess each successive question. (See Unit 7 for effective test-taking strategy.)

Sources

1. After Johnson, D., & Blalock, J. (1982). Problems of mathematics in children with language disorders. In J. L. Northern (Ed.), *Review manual for speech, language and hearing* (p. 318). Philadelphia, PA: W.B. Saunders.
2. Calvert, D. (1982). Articulation and hearing impairment. In J. L. Northern (Ed.), *Review manual for speech, language and hearing* (p. 232). Philadelphia, PA: W.B. Saunders.
3. After Johnston, J. (1982). The language disordered child. In J. L. Northern (Ed.), *Review manual for speech, language and hearing* (p. 286). Philadelphia, PA: W.B. Saunders.
4. McReynolds, L., & Elbert, M. (1982). Articulation disorders of unknown etiology and their remediation. In J. L. Northern (Ed.), *Review manual for speech, language and hearing* (p. 214). Philadelphia, PA: W.B. Saunders.
5. Nation, J. (1982). Management of speech and language disorders. In J. L. Northern (Ed.), *Review manual for speech, language and hearing* (p. 146). Philadelphia, PA: W.B. Saunders.
6. Kuehn, D. (1982). Assessment of resonance disorders. In J. L. Northern (Ed.), *Review manual for speech, language and hearing* (p. 171). Philadelphia, PA: W.B. Saunders.
7. After Johnston, J. (1982). The language disordered child. In J. L. Northern (Ed.), *Review manual for speech, language and hearing* (p. 286). Philadelphia, PA: W.B. Saunders.
8. After Murray, T. (1982). Phonation: Assessment. In J. L. Northern (Ed.), *Review manual for speech, language and hearing* (p. 450). Philadelphia, PA: W.B. Saunders.
9. After Johnston, J. (1989). The language disordered child. In J. L. Northern (Ed.), *Study guide for Handbook of Speech-Language Pathology and Audiology* (p. 98). Philadelphia, PA: B.C. Decker.
10. Guyette, T., & Baumgartner, S. (1989). Stuttering in the adult. In J. L. Northern (Ed.), *Study guide for Handbook of Speech-Language Pathology and Audiology* (p. 168). Philadelphia, PA: B.C. Decker.
11. Thompson, C. (1989). Articulation disorders in the child with neurogenic pathology. In J. L. Northern (Ed.), *Study guide for Handbook of Speech-Language Pathology and Audiology* (p. 141). Philadelphia, PA: B.C. Decker.

12. Wall, M. (1989). Dysfluency in the child. In J. L. Northern (Ed.), *Study guide for Handbook of Speech-Language Pathology and Audiology* (p. 160). Philadelphia, PA: B.C. Decker.
13. Thompson, C. (1989). Articulation disorders in the child with neurogenic pathology. In J. L. Northern (Ed.), *Study guide for Handbook of Speech-Language Pathology and Audiology* (p. 143). Philadelphia, PA: B.C. Decker.
14. Hegde, M. (1989). Principles of management and remediation. After Johnston, J. The language disordered child. In J. L. Northern (Ed.), *Study guide for Handbook of Speech-Language Pathology and Audiology* (p. 99). Philadelphia, PA: B.C. Decker.

UNIT 9

GUESSING

Directions for the Praxis encourage guessing to increase performance. You may recall that previously there was a penalty for guessing, and examinees were encouraged to leave questions blank to avoid having points subtracted. Recent revisions to the Praxis, however, score only correct answers. No points are subtracted for wrong answers. Therefore, guessing is likely to increase your performance.

Effective guessing is an essential test-taking strategy. Each Praxis Examination question contains five answer choices. Even a wild guess provides you with a 1 in 5 chance of selecting the correct answer. Effective guessing involves increasing this 1 in 5 chance to an even greater probability.

If you know nothing about the question, take a wild guess. Fill in any answer bubble. If you have at least some information about the question, eliminate as many answer choices as possible and choose among the remaining choices. As you eliminate choices, this technique increases the probability of selecting the correct answer from 1 in 5, as for a wild guess, to perhaps 1 in 4 or 1 in 3, depending on the number of choices you are able to eliminate.

There are effective ways of making guesses for questions that you might otherwise skip. The most effective technique for guessing for questions you do not reach is to avoid random selection. Random selection of answer choices decreases your probability of adding additional points to your score. You can demonstrate this probability for yourself. Take a sheet of paper, and number it from 1 through 20. Beside each number write in random fashion either A, B, C, D, or E. Now lay the sheet aside and repeat the procedure on another different sheet. Compare the two sheets. Upon comparison of your answers, you will note that some answers match merely by chance.

Next, choose your one favorite letter from A to E. Prepare another sheet with the same letter for each of the 20 slots. Note the frequency that your letter occurs on the original list. If you always choose your favorite letter for questions you do not reach you will probably be correct much more often than choosing randomly among all five letters. Therefore, if time is called before you have finished, select one letter and fill in *only* this letter in the remaining response bubbles on your answer sheet.

Practice this strategy with the following set of questions. Use two separate sheets of paper for the first two exercises, then use the space provided below each question for the final exercise. First, without reading the questions, fill in the answers using random selection of either A, B, C, D, or E. Next, choose your favorite letter and use it to fill in the answer spaces. Finally, complete the examination by reading and answering each question and by guessing for the questions you do not know. Compare your results on each of these exercises to the correct answers.

1. Objective voice evaluation includes such factors as[1]

   A. precise respiratory and phonatory measures
   B. ratings of vocal severity
   C. results of standardized test protocols
   D. calibrated audiological findings
   E. perceptual description of the voice

Answer ________

2. Developmental learning skills are those response systems that[2]

   A. cannot be taught or experimentally manipulated
   B. serve as prerequisites for the developmental process
   C. serve as the basis for teaching programs
   D. are used to generate motor behavior
   E. are unique to language acquisition

Answer ________

3. In Spanish-influenced English, the production of "Juan left yesterday. I think is coming back tomorrow" is due to[3]

   A. the operation of a morphological rule
   B. the operation of a stylistic rule
   C. the operation of a syntactic rule
   D. the operation of a phonological rule
   E. narrative style

Answer ________

4. Measurement of speech and language disorders implies[4]

   A. only the use of "formal" testing instruments
   B. descriptions of both causal factors and symptoms
   C. the use of quantitative data over qualitative data
   D. focus on behavioral description
   E. developing a battery of tests that measures all aspects of speech and language

Answer ________

5. Generalization is viewed as[5]

   A. a natural sequel to the teaching program
   B. a product of an effective measurement system
   C. a function of the teacher
   D. a function of the clinician
   E. a skill to be taught by the school and home

Answer ________

6. Behaviors that result in excessive muscular tension in the vocal tract are known as[6]

   A. glottal fry behaviors
   B. functional laryngitis
   C. hyperfunctional behaviors
   D. peristaltic behaviors
   E. fatigue factor behaviors

Answer ________

7. A fact NOT considered to be important when selecting a sound inventory is[7]

   A. sample adequacy
   B. normative data
   C. number of years the test has been in use
   D. material presentation
   E. scoring and analysis procedures

Answer ________

8. The acoustic reinforcement of particular components of the sound generated at the larynx by dynamic changes in the shape of the vocal tract is referred to as[8]

   A. phonation
   B. prosody
   C. speech
   D. resonation
   E. palatal insufficiency

Answer ________

9. Which of the following statements is NOT true?[9]

   A. Fundamental frequency and intensity are related to pitch and loudness, respectively
   B. Intensity is determined by subglottal air pressure
   C. Fundamental frequency is determined by glottal state and transglottal pressure differential
   D. Fundamental frequency and intensity are related to loudness and pitch, respectively
   E. Intensity is determined by the degree of constriction and length of the subglottal vocal tract

Answer ________

10. Which of the following is NOT characteristic of children with dyskinetic dysarthria?[10]

   A. Movement patterns in impaired muscle groups are lacking in coordination
   B. Speech production is mildly impaired
   C. All four extremities are often involved and, therefore, the label quadriplegia is sometimes applied
   D. Involuntary movement of impaired muscle groups may be seen
   E. Variability exists in speech production

Answer ________

Answers

1. (A), 2. (B), 3. (C), 4. (B), 5. (E), 6. (C), 7. (C), 8. (D), 9. (D), 10. (D)

Sources

1. Johnson, T., & Child, D. (1989). Voice disorders in the child. In J. L. Northern (Ed.), *Study guide for Handbook of Speech-Language Pathology and Audiology* (p. 215). Philadelphia, PA: B.C. Decker.
2. Turton, L. (1982). Communication and language instruction for severely handicapped children and youth. In J. L. Northern (Ed.), *Review manual for speech, language and hearing* (p. 317). Philadelphia, PA: W.B. Saunders.
3. Payne, K. (1989). Speech and language differences and disorders of multicultural populations. In J. L. Northern (Ed.), *Study guide for Handbook of Speech-Language Pathology and Audiology* (p. 269). Philadelphia, PA: B.C. Decker.
4. Nation, J. (1982). Management of speech and language disorders. In J. L. Northern (Ed.), *Review manual for speech, language and hearing* (p. 414). Philadelphia, PA: W.B. Saunders.
5. Turton, L. (1982). Communication and language instruction for severely handicapped children and youth. In J. L. Northern (Ed.), *Review manual for speech, language and hearing* (p. 318). Philadelphia, PA: W.B. Saunders.
6. Johnson, T., & Child, D. (1982). Voice disorders in the child. In J. L. Northern (Ed.), *Review manual for speech, language and hearing* (p. 215). Philadelphia, PA: W.B. Saunders.
7. Bankson, N., & Bernthal, J. (1982). Articulation assessment. In J. L. Northern (Ed.), *Review manual for speech, language and hearing* (p. 204). Philadelphia, PA: W.B. Saunders.
8. Guilford, A. (1989). Language disorders in the adolescent. In J. L. Northern (Ed.), *Study guide for Handbook of Speech-Language Pathology and Audiology* (p. 195). Philadelphia, PA: B.C. Decker.
9. Payne, K. Original material.
10. Thompson, C. (1989). Articulation disorders in the child with neurogenic pathology. In J. L. Northern (Ed.), *Study guide for Handbook of Speech-Language Pathology and Audiology* (p. 142). Philadelphia, PA: B.C. Decker.

APPENDIX

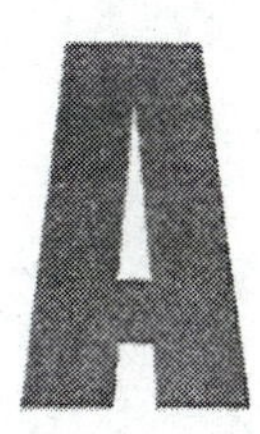

ARE YOU PREPARED FOR THE PRAXIS?

Appendix B contains a simulated Praxis examination. Test your preparation for the Praxis by answering the following questions. The values for each answer are given. When you have completed this form, total the points for each question and refer to the score values at the end of the questionnaire for your scoring analysis.

NO	MAYBE	YES	
0 [ ]	1 [ ]	2 [ ]	1. Have you read all pertinent information in the Praxis Bulletin?
0 [ ]	0 [ ]	1 [ ]	2. Are you familiar with the date and time of the examination?
0 [ ]	1 [ ]	2 [ ]	3. Are you familiar with format, instructions, and areas covered by the examination?
1 [ ]	2 [ ]	3 [ ]	4. Have you reviewed the coursework necessary for the examination?
1 [ ]	2 [ ]	3 [ ]	5. Have you studied material from courses you have not taken?
1 [ ]	2 [ ]	3 [ ]	6. Have you studied the areas of the examination that are most difficult for you?
1 [ ]	2 [ ]	3 [ ]	7. Have you reviewed undergraduate coursework?

0 [ ]	0 [ ]	1 [ ]	8. Do you know the recommendation for guessing on the examination?
0 [ ]	1 [ ]	2 [ ]	9. Have you read the ASHA Code of Ethics?
1 [ ]	2 [ ]	3 [ ]	10. Are you confident of your knowledge?
0 [ ]	1 [ ]	2 [ ]	11. Have you released negative thoughts about the examination?
0 [ ]	1 [ ]	2 [ ]	12. Have you adopted the appropriate positive mental outlook?
2 [ ]	4 [ ]	6 [ ]	13. Have you practiced with questions similar to those on the examination?
2 [ ]	4 [ ]	6 [ ]	14. Have you exercised the necessary cognitive requirements for answering the type of questions on the examination?
1 [ ]	2 [ ]	3 [ ]	15. Can you answer most questions in less than 38 seconds?
0 [ ]	1 [ ]	2 [ ]	16. Can you implement the necessary stress reduction activities?
0 [ ]	1 [ ]	2 [ ]	17. Can you postpone concern about other worries in your life and focus on the examination?
1 [ ]	2 [ ]	3 [ ]	18. Do you possess a high level of motivation to perform as well as you probably can?
2 [ ]	4 [ ]	6 [ ]	19. Are you able to make accurate and appropriate clinical judgments about clients?

2 [ ]	4 [ ]	6 [ ]	20. Are you able to make applications of theory or facts to real-life or hypothetical situations?
2 [ ]	4 [ ]	6 [ ]	21. Can you factor out pertinent details of a clinical case to make appropriate conclusions?
2 [ ]	4 [ ]	6 [ ]	22. Can you derive relationships among details and draw clear conclusions?
0 [ ]	3 [ ]	6 [ ]	23. Did you score high on other standardized tests, e.g., SAT, GRE?
1 [ ]	2 [ ]	3 [ ]	24. Does your reasoning reflect the attitudes, values, current practices, and professional standards of the profession?
1 [ ]	2 [ ]	3 [ ]	25. Can you sublimate your personal beliefs in favor of the consensus of the profession?
2 [ ]	4 [ ]	6 [ ]	26. Have you successfully exercised the reasoning skills involved in answering the type of questions on the examination?
1 [ ]	2 [ ]	3 [ ]	27. Do you fully understand material when it is read quickly?
1 [ ]	2 [ ]	3 [ ]	28. Does your academic and clinical background provide an adequate basis for understanding the intricacies of the questions on the examination?
1 [ ]	2 [ ]	3 [ ]	29. Can you interpret charts and graphs and make appropriate conclusions?

1	2	3	
[ ]	[ ]	[ ]	30. Are you familiar with the various research designs?
1	2	3	
[ ]	[ ]	[ ]	31. Can you identify a type of research design given a description of a method?
1	2	3	
[ ]	[ ]	[ ]	32. Can you identify dependent and independent variables in a research study?
2	4	6	
[ ]	[ ]	[ ]	33. Are you familiar with proven test-taking strategies?
2	4	6	
[ ]	[ ]	[ ]	34. Have you exercised individual test-taking strategies with success?
2	4	6	
[ ]	[ ]	[ ]	35. Are you familiar with the rule for answering a set number of questions per time block?
0	3	6	
[ ]	[ ]	[ ]	36. Can you answer the practice examination with at least 60 percent accuracy?
0	1	2	
[ ]	[ ]	[ ]	37. Do you recognize the importance of rest and appropriate nutrition on your performance?
2	4	6	
[ ]	[ ]	[ ]	38. Have you given maximum effort toward preparation for the examination?

Scoring Analysis

37–63	**Not prepared—Review coursework and test preparation skills**
64–89	**Not prepared—Review test preparation skills**
90–116	**Minimally prepared**
117–142	**Well prepared**

APPENDIX

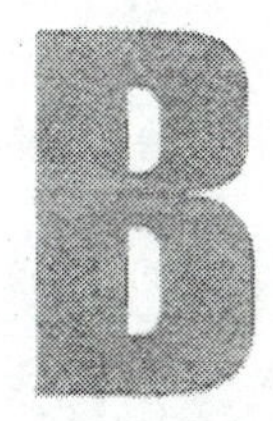

PRACTICE TEST FOR THE PRAXIS IN SPEECH-LANGUAGE PATHOLOGY

Answer all of the questions in the corresponding space on the Answer Sheet. Record the current time in the space below. Do not exceed 2 hours. If you finish before 2 hours, go back and recheck your answers.

SHOULD YOU GUESS? Scoring the Practice Test involves counting correct answers only. Blank spaces are counted as wrong answers. Therefore, you should fill in a response for every question, even if you must guess.

When you have completed the Practice Test, compare your answers to the correct answers. Count each correct answer as one point, then tally your raw score. Compare your raw score to the Conversion Table to estimate your Praxis score.

TIME NOW: ________

PRAXIS—SPEECH-LANGUAGE PATHOLOGY

Time—120 minutes
150 questions

Directions: Each of the questions or incomplete statements below is followed by five suggested answers or completions. Select the one that is best in each case and then fill in the corresponding lettered space on the answer sheet with a heavy, dark mark so that you cannot see the letter.

1. During assessment, reliability of clinical observations is ultimately important because

   A. test results cannot be interpreted without it
   B. test manuals suggest one obtain it
   C. the tester has more confidence in the consistency of the results
   D. clinical decisions are based on accuracy of the tester's perceptions
   E. it means the tester has done everything properly

2. A clinician wishes to evaluate the effectiveness of a treatment method on clients. The best indicator of the success of the treatment would be

   A. the changes in behavior that result from the treatment
   B. the degree to which clients display interest and enthusiasm for the treatment
   C. the amount of time that it takes for clients to show improvement
   D. the number of trials until clients experience success with the treatment
   E. the consistency of the client's response

3. A researcher sent out a questionnaire to measure the attitudes of stutterers toward speaking situations. The questionnaire asked stutters to respond to items such as "My wife makes telephone calls on my behalf" with response options of Always, Usually, Infrequently, Rarely, or Never. This type of scale is known as

   A. Ordinal
   B. Frequency
   C. Nominal
   D. Ratio
   E. Continuous

4. A researcher evaluated the results of a treatment procedure for stuttering. Performance of 5 subjects was measured 4 times before starting treatment, then the treatment was conducted for 3 months. Finally the researcher took 4 more measures of performance in the absence of treatment. This kind of research design is known as

   A. Static Group Comparison Design
   B. Single Group Time Series Design
   C. Single Treatment Counterbalance Design
   D. Crossover Design
   E. One Group Pretest-Post-test Design

5. Elements of the diagnostic report include all of the following EXCEPT

   A. Short-term goals of therapy
   B. Background information
   C. Test results
   D. Recommended treatment
   E. Impressions

6. Which of the following statements is inappropriate for a diagnostic report?

   A. James has moderately severe hypernasality and a mild articulation disorder caused by velopharyngeal insufficiency

B. Kent's diagnosis of minimal brain dysfunction is supported by a history of seizures and an abnormal electroencephalogram
C. Hal has complete aphonia following total laryngectomy on May 27, 1988
D. While the examiner cannot interpret his behavior, Ed's reference to violence in all his responses is a serious concern
E. Dennis' difficulty with expressive language is the direct result of his mother's overprotection and serious emotional problems

7. A 4-year-old child is referred for evaluation of dysfluency. Behavioral characteristics consist of 3 syllable repetitions per 100 words, word and phrase repetitions, and revision of utterances. It is reported that his maternal uncle and grandfather also stutter. The most appropriate courses of action for therapy is

A. recommend parent counseling and reevaluate after 6 months
B. recommend parent counseling and begin therapy to reinforce fluency
C. administer direct behavior modification therapy focused on stuttered syllables and words
D. delay therapy until the child enters school but monitor every 6 months
E. conduct desensitizing techniques aimed at specific conditions under which dysfluencies occur

8. The literature documents several cases of children who failed to learn language due to complete lack of human contact and linguistic stimulation. The position that children learn language naturally at a very early age, after which language learning is difficult or impossible, is known as

A. innateness hypothesis
B. motherese hypothesis
C. critical age hypothesis
D. functional core hypothesis
E. strong cognitive theory

9. According to ASHA's position on social dialects, which of the following is the appropriate intervention for speakers of non-standard English?

A. Mandatory clinical intervention to teach standard English
B. Speech therapy should be provided in the native dialect
C. Speech pathologists may provide elective clinical services to dialect speakers
D. The dialect should be treated as a communication disorder and eradicated
E. Speech pathologists should not provide clinical intervention for dialect speakers

10. A 3-year-old boy articulates "fumb" for thumb, "wabbit" for rabbit, and "duce" for juice. The most appropriate advice to the parents is

A. recommend to an audiologist for hearing evaluation
B. enroll him in speech clinic for articulation therapy
C. ignore these behaviors since they are developmentally appropriate
D. seek a complete speech and language evaluation
E. recommend home exercises to correct error sounds

11. A speech production which is the result of deficient motor programming or sensorimotor impairment is

A. dysarthria
B. ataxia
C. aphasia
D. agraphia
E. apraxia

12. During the case history interview, the mother of a language-learning disabled child

states that she caused her child's disability because she drank three beers to ease labor pain. Which of the following replies by the clinician is most appropriate?

A. "While your action was not good, you did not cause your child's disability."
B. "Don't blame yourself. It can happen to anyone."
C. "I know you feel badly, but I can help your child."
D. "We don't know exactly what causes language-learning disabilities."
E. "That was in the past. Now let's focus on your child's ability."

13. The stages of Piaget's development that are most crucial to language development are

A. concrete operations and formal operations
B. concrete operations and preoperational
C. concrete operations and sensorimotor
D. sensorimotor and preoperational
E. preoperational and concrete operational

14. Prior to providing treatment a clinician provides a naturalistic environment and counts the frequency of misarticulations in a client with a lateral lisp. This activity is known as

A. probe
B. baseline
C. pretest
D. language sample
E. shaping

15. In the perception of speech, the acoustic identification and discrimination of vowels is primarily due to

A. formant frequencies
B. formant bandwidth
C. voice onset time
D. F_0 to F_1 transition
E. F_1 to F_2 transition

16. Which of the following errors most negatively affects intelligibility of persons with a severe hearing loss?

A. Substitution of vowels
B. Errors involving voice-voiceless confusion
C. Substitution of nasals for stops
D. Omission of final consonants
E. Inappropriate relationships between stressed and unstressed syllables

17. Which of the following should be considered for a high-end electronic communication device with synthesized speech?

A. A 10-year-old child with mild language delay and a moderate articulation disorder
B. A 12-year-old deaf child
C. A 6-year-old mentally retarded girl with a language age of 1.0 who primarily relies on gestures
D. A 51-year-old man with mild motor problems who uses manual signs and gestures
E. A 4-year-old hard-of-hearing child who is learning oral communication

18. A young child is referred for a speech and language evaluation. Following the case history medical report the clinician immediately suspects that the child may have a hearing impairment. Which of the following indicators is most likely the reason for this suspicion?

A. Physical developmental milestones were normal, but the child ceased babbling at 8 months
B. Compared to older siblings, the child's developmental history showed marked delays and one parent has a hearing loss
C. The child's mother was exposed to rubella during the eighth month of pregnancy
D. The child had otitis media at 9 months
E. The child has had several high fevers accompanied by congestion

19. A 6-year-old child who says *tee* for *see*, *tack* for *sack*, but *soo* for *shoe* exhibits a disorder of

A. phoneme production
B. auditory reception
C. word retrieval
D. phonological process
E. delayed language development

20. The Yawn-Sigh approach is most effective for individuals with which of the following?

A. Conversion aphonia
B. Ventricular fold phonation
C. Spastic dysphonia
D. Vocal nodules
E. Vocal hyperfunction

21. Which of the following articulatory errors would have the greatest effect on speech intelligibility of a child with repaired velopharyngeal incompetency?

A. A continual nasal snort
B. Pharyngeal fricatives
C. Glottal articulations
D. Phonemic omissions
E. Posterior nasal fricatives

22. A characteristic of autistic children that is NOT found in mentally retarded children is

I. normal to high intelligence
II. failure to develop social skills
III. overreaction to sensory stimuli
IV. delayed language development

A. I only
B. I and II
C. II and III
D. III and IV
E. IV only

23. A test instrument is administered to a client by two different examiners. If the two scores achieved by the client are the same, the test is presumed to have

A. construct validity
B. predictive validity
C. content validity
D. inter-rater reliability
E. split-half reliability

24. Which of the following is a secondary reinforcer?

A. Raisins are presented to a mentally retarded child for a correct response
B. Verbal praise is given to an adult stutterer for each minute of sustained fluency
C. A clinician says "stop" to a stutterer to interrupt a repetition
D. The level of white noise is lowered in response to fluent speech for a stutterer
E. A child is allowed to engage in play time after therapy

25. When a behavior is mastered in therapy and used properly in the natural environment, it is said to be

A. extinguished
B. discriminated
C. maintained
D. generalized
E. carried over

26. A procedure to assess carryover is known as

A. probe
B. shaping
C. fading
D. modeling
E. scaffolding

27. A clinician wishes to train the production of /l/. The client is instructed to (1) protrude the tongue, (2) elevate the tongue, (3) place the tongue in alveolar position, (4) flap the tongue. Each successive step is reinforced. The technique is known as

A. instructions
B. prompts
C. fading
D. shaping
E. scaffolding

28. Which of the following is NOT a syntactic feature of African-American English?

A. copula deletion
B. habitual "be"
C. multiple negatives
D. omission of articles
E. s-plural deletion

29. During therapy the clinician notices that a 6-year-old child tends to lose attention and play with the buttons on his shirt. The clinician tells the child that he will receive a lollipop at the end of the session if he continues to concentrate and avoids playing with his buttons. This reinforcement method is known as

A. differential reinforcement of incompatible behavior
B. differential reinforcement of alternative behavior
C. differential reinforcement of low rates of responding
D. negative reinforcement of an undesirable behavior
E. positive reinforcement of an undesirable behavior

30. A test is biased if

A. no one can achieve a perfect score
B. most individuals fail the test
C. one population achieves consistently high scores
D. a discrepancy exists in performance for a certain population
E. it is not administered according to the test manual

31. Which of the following characterizes language development in severely mentally retarded children?

I. Slow to develop language
II. Children eventually catch up to their peers
III. More delay with certain features than with others
IV. Children may learn in different ways

A. I and II only
B. I, II, and III
C. II and IV only
D. I, III, and IV
E. II, III, and IV

32. Which of the following is a true statement concerning Standard English?

I. It is not a dialect
II. It is the written version
III. It is preferred for common social interactions
IV. It is the only correct way to speak

A. I and II
B. I, II, and III
C. II, III, and IV
D. II and III
E. III and IV

33. A language test that requests children to point to the picture which represents "Mommy gave the ball to her" is most probably examining

A. verbal expression
B. semantic relations
C. vocabulary level
D. auditory reception
E. word associations

34. Which of the following indicates that a 12-month-old child is in the holophrastic stage?

A. a child says "eh" and reaches for her bottle
B. a child points to a picture and says "was dat?"
C. a child points to her eyes in response to "Show me eyes."
D. a child finishes her drink and says "duce" indicating more juice
E. a child points to the cat and says "kitty"

35. When a 3-year-old child says "Daddy goed away" this is an indication of

A. a semantic error
B. syntactic ambiguity
C. generalization of a morphological rule
D. a syntactic error
E. phonological process

36. A 63-year-old male sustained a cerebral vascular accident resulting in ataxic dysarthria. Most likely the damage was incurred in which area of the brain?

    A. cerebellum
    B. brainstem
    C. temporal lobe
    D. frontal lobe
    E. occipital lobe

37. Although many clients have similar disorder characteristics, an individual treatment plan is desirable according to each client's specific needs. Which of the following is of greatest value for the success of any treatment method?

    A. The clinician's ability to implement the procedures
    B. The theoretical orientation and supporting research from which the method is derived
    C. The activities and materials that support the method
    D. The amount of structure inherent in the method
    E. Applicability of the method for a wide range of clients

38. Diagnostic procedures involve several basic processes. Which of the following is not a goal of diagnosis?

    A. Describing symptomatology
    B. Understanding the causal basis for the disorder
    C. Validating the test instruments
    D. Classifying or labeling the disorder
    E. Providing intervention recommendations

39. A 6-year-old child with normal hearing acuity makes the following sound substitutions in initial, medial, and final word positions: t/s; d/z. In a spontaneous speech sample, assimilation errors across words in connected speech rendered speech occasionally unintelligible and there was limited stimulability for s and z, particularly in initial word position. The primary goal for articulation therapy should be to

    A. establish accurate production of /s/ and /z/ in initial position
    B. establish accurate production of /s/ in initial, medial, and final word positions
    C. establish accurate production of /s/ and /z/ in isolation
    D. establish accurate production of /s/ and /z/ in syllables
    E. establish accurate discrimination of /s/ and /z/ from error production in words

40. Which of the following has the least effect on articulation errors?

    A. Diadochokinetic rate
    B. Tongue thrust
    C. Intelligence
    D. Hearing loss
    E. Absence of dentition

41. Taunisha is a 3-year-old African-American child referred for speech and language services. Case history reveals chronic otitis media; however, hearing is normal bilaterally. She has a limited vocabulary and absence of grammatical morphemes. Multiple articulation errors include final consonant omission, stopping, unstressed syllable omission, gliding, and cluster simplification. Her speech is moderately intelligible, but her parents are able to interpret. The most accurate description of Taunisha's ability is

    A. normal language development process
    B. normal language development with dialect features
    C. phonological disorder without dialect features
    D. phonological disorder with dialect features
    E. language disorder with dialect features

42. Which of the following is NOT a goal of phonological sample analysis?

A. To examine perceptual abilities
B. To obtain a phonetic inventory
C. To sample emerging phonemes
D. To examine frequency characteristics of error sounds
E. To supplement standardized instruments

43. Which of the following is an instrument that analyzes all aspects of articulation of single words?

A. Kahn-Lewis Phonological Analysis
B. Fisher-Logemann Test of Articulation Competence
C. Goldman-Fristoe Test of Articulation
D. Arizona Articulation Proficiency Scale
E. Bankson-Bernthal Test of Phonology

44. Phonological disorders are distinguished from articulation disorders in that phonological disorders are

A. disturbances in motoric function
B. linguistic deficits
C. structural anomalies
D. neurological disorders
E. receptive deficits

45. A child with a noticeable and persistent tongue thrust would most probably have difficulty articulating which of the following sounds?

A. /w/
B. /s/
C. /k/
D. /j/
E. /i/

46. Which of the following areas might present difficulty to a school-age child with specific language impairment?

A. Sentence assembly
B. Visuospatial ability
C. Emotional function
D. Abstract reasoning
E. Temporal orientation

47. The emergence of literacy is intimately related to receptive and expressive language abilities. Thus, children with language learning disabilities are at risk for difficulty in reading achievement. Impairment to which of the following is the best indicator of pending reading difficulty?

A. Sequential memory
B. Vocabulary development
C. Metaphonological ability
D. Visual memory
E. Symbolic meaning

48. Which of the following is the most important consideration in selecting aided versus unaided augmentative communication systems?

A. Cost effectiveness
B. Iconicity of symbols
C. Level of language development
D. Degree of motor control of upper extremities
E. Intelligence

49. Under which condition is it permissible for a clinician to release client records to another professional?

A. Only if the professional requests in writing
B. Only with the knowledge of the client or guardian
C. Only with the written consent of the client or guardian
D. Always when the client is referred to the professional
E. Only if the records have significant bearing on the client treatment

50. Which of the following is true of transformational rules?

A. They change the sentence from a declarative to an interrogative
B. They dictate syntactical word order
C. They render sentences ungrammatical

D. They change words to another syntactic category
E. They differentiate ambiguity

51. Two-year-old Gary has been referred for clinical services after surgery to repair his bilateral cleft lip and palate. What is the first procedure that should be done by the speech-language pathologist?

A. Outline specific goals for therapy
B. Assess speech and language capabilities
C. Examine oral structure and assess muscular function
D. Obtain a baseline description of articulatory accuracy
E. Conduct activities to stimulate motor function

52. In the process of normal aging, in-class word substitutions and word retrieval difficulties are observed. Calling a calculator a computer is a linguistic error due to

A. lexical ambiguity
B. redundancy rule
C. structural ambiguity
D. subcategorization
E. semantic properties

53. Morphemes that change verbs to nouns such as "ation" as in *preparation* are known as

A. free morphemes
B. productive morphemes
C. derivational morphemes
D. inflectional morphemes
E. root morphemes

54. Saying "aks" for "ask" is a predictable dialectal modification known as

A. contraction
B. metathesis
C. assimilation
D. redundancy reduction
E. regularization

55. Localized mass lesions to the vocal folds such as nodules, polyps, or cysts may result in all of the following EXCEPT

A. hoarseness
B. breathiness
C. tremors
D. hyponasality
E. hypernasality

56. Pragmatic rules include which of the following?

I. Turn taking
II. Eye behavior
III. Gestures
IV. Initiating conversation

A. I, II, and III
B. II and III
C. I and IV
D. I only
E. I, II, and IV

57. An adolescent boy exhibits auditory processing and short-term memory deficits, word finding difficulties, and deficits in verbal reasoning and planning. His teacher reports that he lacks social communication, especially in using language for jokes, sarcasm, and figurative language. Which of the following processes is most probably affected?

A. Functional communication
B. Pragmatic ability
C. Metalinguistic ability
D. Paralinguistic ability
E. Strategic language use

58. "Can you please pass the salt?" is an example of

A. sarcasm
B. direct speech act
C. indirect speech act
D. idiom
E. presupposition

59. The Education for All Handicapped Act (P.L. 94-142) mandated free and appropriate education in the least restrictive environment for children with disabilities. Which of the following conditions complies with this mandate?

A. A child with a profound hearing loss is educated in an oral-aural school for the deaf
B. A child with Attention Deficit Hyperactivity Disorder receives instruction in a special education classroom
C. A preschool child with cerebral palsy attends a Head Start program
D. All children with language learning disabilities receive instruction in a self-contained classroom environment
E. A child with Specific Language Disability is placed in the special education program

60. Research and best practice have firmly established that early intervention is mandatory for infants and toddlers who are experiencing developmental delays in cognitive development, physical development, speech and language development, and/or psychosocial development. Required services include a multidisciplinary assessment and family-centered intervention approaches. These services are mandated by which of the following laws?

A. ADA
B. IDEA
C. P.L. 94-142
D. P.L. 99-457, Part B
E. P.L. 99-457, Part H

61. An example of a criterion referenced measure is

A. Mean length of utterance
B. Stanford-Binet Test of Intelligence
C. Peabody Picture Vocabulary Test
D. Test of Language Development—I2
E. Clinical Evaluation of Language Fundamentals

62. A 4-year-old preschool child is slow to develop socially, emotionally, and cognitively. Following a full battery of tests, her intelligence quotient is determined to be 68, which is 2 standard deviations below the mean. Her intellectual ability is classified as

A. profound
B. severe
C. moderate
D. mild
E. normal

63. In the determination of the prognosis for a 5-year-old boy with a language disability sustained as a result of traumatic brain injury, the best prognostic indicator of success of treatment is

A. socioeconomic status
B. length of spontaneous recovery
C. age of onset
D. extent and locus of injury
E. the combined number of risk factors

64. Specific language impairment is a significant deficit in language ability without concomitant deficits in cognition or motoric or psychological domains. The most notable language characteristic of children with specific language impairment is

A. limited use of vocabulary and grammatical morphemes
B. inability to follow instructions
C. echolalia
D. use of gestures
E. idiosyncratic use of language

65. A 6-year-old child who has sustained a head injury from a fall from playground equipment may exhibit which of the following?

A. Disturbances in reading and writing
B. Impairments of attention, perception, and memory
C. Errors of symbolic representation
D. Difficulty in processing information
E. Inefficient word retrieval ability

66. An investigator wishes to test the hypothesis that stuttering, if left untreated, becomes progressively more severe, particularly during adolescence. In order to conduct a developmental study, the methodology should include

    A. comparing the prevalence of severe stuttering in a group of eighth graders
    B. surveying speech-language pathologists about severe stutterers across all grades
    C. administering a severity rating scale to a group of stuttering clients selected at random from all grades
    D. administering a severity rating scale to a group of adolescent stutterers
    E. surveying adult stutterers about the progression of their symptoms

67. A team of researchers conducts a longitudinal study of high-risk infants from birth through adolescence. They measure the same subjects periodically on a number of variables including language development, academic achievement, physical growth, and social-emotional adjustment. This type of research is best known as

    A. ex post facto
    B. experimental
    C. historical
    D. developmental
    E. correlational

68. In a study focusing on infant discrimination between auditory stimuli, an investigator presents various pure tone signals to 30 infants between 3 and 6 months of age, and observes the changes in their sucking reflex responses. In this study, sucking response is

    A. an intervening variable
    B. the dependent variable
    C. the organismic variable
    D. the reactive measure
    E. the independent variable

69. A third grade teacher is concerned that one of her pupils speaks with excessive rate and appears to have a mild articulation disorder. He is also observed to have a short attention span, disorganized thought processes, and lack of synchrony between thought, language, and speech. The speech-language pathologist should suspect which of the following?

    A. Cluttering dysfluency
    B. Functional articulation disorder
    C. Learning disability
    D. Language delay
    E. Emotional disturbance

70. Which of the following is the best criterion to determine when a child should be dismissed from therapy?

    A. When speech is 90% intelligible in the therapy session
    B. After the preestablished number of sessions has been conducted
    C. At the end of the school year
    D. When parents and teachers feel that therapy is no longer warranted
    E. When all goals have been reached at the established criterion level

71. During assessment for a phonological disorder the clinician provides modeling with visual and physical cues for production of the child's error sounds. It is exhibited that the child can make some correct productions of error sounds. The child's ability to imitate correct productions of error sound is indicative of

    A. phonological awareness
    B. phonological discrimination
    C. phonological organization
    D. phonetic perception
    E. cognitive ability

72. Phonation with incomplete closure of the ventricular folds would create which of the following vocal characteristics?

    A. Hoarseness
    B. Aphonia
    C. Breathiness
    D. Hyponasality
    E. Breathy-hoarse

73. Joseph is a second grade boy who is extremely active and involved in all sports. His mother reports that he is the youngest child and he is competitive with his two older brothers. Use of his voice in screaming and yelling has resulted in a vocal quality that is characterized by hoarseness. A laryngeal examination should focus on locating a protrusion on the vocal folds at which location?

    A. Unilaterally at the cartilaginous portion
    B. Unilaterally at the membranous portion
    C. Unilaterally at the midpoint
    D. Bilaterally at the midpoint
    E. Bilaterally at the anterior middle thirds

74. A child who scores normally on nonverbal tests of intelligence but fails to establish the social relationships necessary for language learning is most probably

    A. mentally deficient
    B. emotionally disturbed
    C. autistic
    D. language learning disabled
    E. minimally brain dysfunctional

75. Which quality of speech would be the result of velopharyngeal insufficiency?

    A. Hypernasality
    B. Hyponasality
    C. Nasal snort
    D. Nasal twang
    E. Breathiness

76. Which of the following conditions is most common among children 4 to 6 years of age?

    A. Vocal nodules
    B. Papilloma
    C. Cysts
    D. Polyps
    E. Contact ulcers

77. The source of the sound vibration necessary for esophageal speech is

    A. esophagus
    B. trachea
    C. pharynx
    D. pharyngeo-esophageal segment
    E. epiglottis

78. Which of the following is NOT a crucial element in the evaluation of vocal function?

    A. Intensity
    B. Pitch
    C. Voice quality
    D. Resonance
    E. Vocal range

79. A 24-year-old woman is referred for vocal rehabilitation. No medical rehabilitation is warranted and the client is counseled to exercise vocal rest for 10 days and to seek a program for smoking cessation. After the appropriate time period the clinician finds no improvement due to failure to follow the prescribed instructions. The most appropriate step is to

    A. initiate relaxation therapy
    B. begin intensive symptomatic therapy
    C. refer for psychological evaluation
    D. investigate the social environment
    E. create interim behavioral adjustments

80. In the process of the medical examination for speech production, several processes involving aerodynamic and radiographic techniques are used. Which of the following allows the viewing and recording of structural movements in the velopharyngeal mechanism?

    A. Videofluorography
    B. Computer assisted tomography (CAT) scans
    C. Endoscopy
    D. Spectrography
    E. Manometry

81. An individual who experiences a traumatic, postlingual hearing loss will most probably experience deterioration in the articulation of which of the following sounds?

A. Stop consonants
B. Final consonants
C. Glides and liquids
D. Front vowels
E. Initial consonants

82. Jack's language functioning was determined to be at the 5.8 age equivalent. Which of the following approaches to measurement was used to describe Jack's performance?

A. Norm-referenced
B. Criterion referenced
C. Client referenced
D. Clinician referenced
E. Group referenced

83. A prognosis is

A. a statement of the cause of the disorder
B. a description of the characteristics of the disorder
C. a plan for rehabilitation of the disorder
D. a statement of the possible outcomes with therapy
E. the maximum achievement level of the client

84. Which of the following is NOT true of African-American English?

A. It is creole derived from English and African languages
B. It is a corruption of Standard English
C. It is comprehensible to other speakers of English
D. It is an orderly, rule-governed variety of English
E. Its features derive from predictable language changes

85. In order to assure that diagnostic reports are understood by parents, and are useful to other professionals, a well-written report should

A. avoid all technical jargon
B. fully describe the child's disabilities and prognosis
C. report only quantifiable data
D. provide an explanatory summary statement
E. make precise recommendations

86. A style of speaking based only on phonological and prosodic differences is

A. dialect
B. accent
C. idiolect
D. pidgin
E. creole

87. The creolist theory of the origin of African-American English posits that

A. it is the misuse of Standard English
B. it derives from mixture of English and African languages
C. it has predictable variations from Standard English
D. it exists because of segregation of African-Americans
E. it shares some features with Old English

88. Which of the following is a FALSE statement concerning dialects?

A. Everyone speaks a dialect
B. Dialects are errors of communication
C. Dialects of a language are mutually intelligible
D. No dialect is better than another
E. Standard English is a dialect

89. A speech-language pathologist finds that there are no test instruments which do not contain biases against her client who is from Daufuske Island, SC and who speaks Gullah. An acceptable alternative would be to

A. select the instrument with the least bias
B. score all items missed as correct
C. modify the test instrument
D. use any test, but mistrust the results
E. use any test since there are no unbiased tests available

90. During the oral examination a clinician observes asymmetry of the lips, deviation of the tongue and uvula to the right side, and a weak gag reflex. The client's speech is also slow, slurred, and monotonic. The clinician should

A. conduct further tests for aphasia
B. examine structures for a submucous cleft
C. assess swallowing response
D. recommend surgery before initiating further examination
E. begin therapy to improve oral motor response

91. In which of the following cases should language therapy be recommended?

A. A 2-year-old child uses gestures and whines for communication
B. A 5.8-year-old child has a language age equivalent of 5.3
C. A 6-year-old child has a mean length of utterance of 4.5
D. An 8-year-old child scores 5 points below the mean and the standard deviation is 10
E. A 4-year-old boy exhibits whole word repetitions

92. Which of the following is NOT an essential consideration in selecting an appropriate language test for an elementary school child?

A. How quickly the test can be administered
B. Whether the test requires classroom type activities
C. Whether the test contains biases for the child's cultural group
D. The nature of the child's disorder
E. How many subtests are included in the test

93. A patient with traumatic brain injury is given the following diagnostic procedures:
SCATBI
WAB
Fluency Rating Scale

Which of the following areas has not been assessed?

A. Auditory discrimination
B. Functional ability
C. Auditory comprehension
D. Naming ability
E. Reasoning ability

94. A 73-year-old man sustained a cerebral vascular accident. Symptoms include general language dysfunction and muscle weakness. Which of the following would indicate that the locus of the lesion is in the right hemisphere?

A. Problems in word retrieval
B. Problems in auditory comprehension
C. Left side neglect
D. Problems in reading and writing
E. Grammatical difficulties

95. A head injury patient who is "Rancho IV" is

A. unresponsive to all stimuli
B. able to respond to commands
C. confused and disoriented
D. able to respond to automatic speech
E. fully responsive but has poor judgment

96. Which of the following instruments is inappropriate for examining right hemisphere dysfunction?

A. MIRBI
B. Test of Visual Neglect
C. RICE
D. SCATBI
E. Revised Token Test

97. Which of the following is a measure of functional communication for adults with neurological disorders?

A. RIPA
B. WAB
C. CADL

D. WNSSP
E. SCATBI

98. A clinician administers an articulation test to a 6-year-old child whose speech is severely unintelligible. The instrument selected by the clinician is designed to examine each error phoneme in distinct phonological contexts such as before and after a number of different phonemes. The instrument used by the clinician is the

A. Bankson-Bernthal Test of Phonology
B. McDonald Deep Test of Articulation
C. Templin-Darley Tests of Articulation
D. Arizona Articulation Proficiency Scale
E. Goldman-Fristoe Test of Articulation

99. A clinician examines a 7-year-old boy for a speech sound disorder. Which of the following is the best indicator for a diagnosis of developmental verbal apraxia rather than a phonological disorder?

A. Presence of substitutions and distortions
B. Absence of oral structural anomalies
C. Automatic recitation tasks have no errors
D. Errors are consistent
E. Consonant cluster reductions

100. During a spontaneous speech exercise a 5-year-old boy says /pwe/ for play and /tʌk/ for truck. The phonological processes exhibited are respectively

A. gliding and backing
B. gliding and cluster reduction
C. backing and cluster reduction
D. backing and gliding
E. cluster reduction and gliding

101. Which of the following is NOT a characteristic of dysarthria?

A. Errors of speech are consistent
B. Muscle tone is weakened
C. Respiration and phonation are affected
D. There are periods of clear speech
E. Severe articulation errors

102. Which of the following is NOT a characteristic of apraxia?

A. Vowels are less affected than consonants
B. Consonants are imprecise
C. Muscle tone is weakened
D. Errors of speech are unpredictable
E. Abnormal prosody

103. Following a stroke, a 68-year-old man displays the following characteristics:

> "Poor articulation marked by unpredictable consonant distortions which become more severe as speaking rate and word complexity increase. The patient's oral examination is unremarkable."

Which of the following would be the most appropriate diagnostic instrument to administer?

A. Apraxia Battery for Adults
B. Frenchay Dysarthria Assessment
C. Porch Index of Communicative Ability
D. Communication Activities of Daily Living
E. Western Aphasia Battery

104. Spoonerisms such as "basketti" for "spaghetti" or "lickstip" for "lipstick" are most characteristic of

A. aphasia
B. anomia
C. apraxia
D. dysarthria
E. phonological disorders

105. Hyperadduction of the vocal folds results in

A. increased intensity
B. breathiness
C. increased pitch
D. decreased pitch
E. hoarseness

106. A speech-language pathologist examines a patient referred for a voice assessment. Results reveal an s/z ratio of 1.35. Which of the following would be a reasonable diagnosis?

A. Conversion aphonia
B. Vocal fold paralysis
C. Vocal polyps
D. Spasmodic dysphonia
E. Infectious laryngitis

107. From the case history information obtained from an adult male with a voice disorder, which of the following categories would be most important in determining a prognosis?

A. Behavioral and environmental factors
B. Medical history of past illnesses and conditions
C. Length of previous voice therapy
D. Onset and course of the disorder
E. Previous test results

108. Which of the following assessment procedures for direct observation in voice assessment allows visual inspection of movement as well as recording?

A. Endoscopy
B. Videoendoscopy
C. Nasometer
D. Visipitch
E. Phonatory function analyzer

109. In distinguishing stuttering from normal dysfluency in a 5-year-old child all of the following can serve to confirm the presence of stuttering EXCEPT

A. high frequency of the dysfluent behavior
B. consistency of the dysfluent behavior
C. presence of whole word repetitions
D. presence of part word repetitions
E. attitude of the parents

110. In the assessment of stuttering the adaptation effect refers to

A. fluent behavior on memorized recitation tasks
B. decreased dysfluent behavior across repeated trials
C. consistent dysfluencies on the same words across repeated trials
D. decreased effectiveness of secondary behaviors in enabling fluency
E. the speaker's psychological adjustment to his disability

111. A speech-language pathologist assesses a 15-year-old boy for an augmentative communication device. The client, who is nonambulatory due to cerebral palsy, is educated in the regular classroom. Which of the following would be the most important consideration in selecting an appropriate communication strategy?

A. Desire for environmental controls
B. The client's communicative and hardware needs
C. Power mobility limitations
D. Teacher's understanding of augmentative devices
E. Degree of acceptability to peers

112. A fluency measurement used for assessing a child's anxiety in several different speaking situations is

A. Stocker Probe Technique
B. Total Dysfluency Index
C. Iowa Scale for Rating Severity of Stuttering
D. Stuttering Prediction Instrument for Young Children
E. Children's Attitude About Talking

113. Which of the following is NOT a major symptom associated with abnormal swallowing?

A. Drooling
B. Flatulence
C. Heartburn
D. Regurgitation
E. Aspiration

114. Which of the following results of the bedside examination for dysphagia would indicate the need for a modified barium swallow procedure?

A. Poor oral control
B. Chewing difficulties
C. Nasal regurgitation
D. Aspiration
E. Food retention in the oral cavity

115. Nasal regurgitation during an abnormal swallow would indicate a problem during which phase of the swallow reaction?

A. Oral preparatory phase
B. Oral phase
C. Pharyngeal phase
D. Esophageal phase
E. Gastric phase

116. Which of the following procedures is the best indicator to determine if a patient is aspirating food into the larynx?

A. Ultrasound
B. Videofiberoptic endoscopy
C. Nasometry
D. Oral motor assessment
E. Bedside examination

117. A 16-year-old boy has been outfitted with a synthesized speech augmentative communication device following recovery from a football accident. His linguistic and operational competencies in using the device are well established. However, it is noted that he refuses to use the device in most situations, giving preference to gestures. Which of the following might be the reason for his refusal?

A. Speed of communication is delayed
B. Use of the device will delay his ability to regain speech skills
C. The device uses picture symbols rather than traditional orthography
D. A limited number of people understand the symbols
E. The device does not allow the use of teenage vernacular

118. In designing an augmentative communication system for a 3-year-old child with both receptive and expressive language deficits, as well as cognitive deficits, the most important consideration for selection of symbol characteristics is

A. transparency iconicity of symbols
B. perceptual distinctiveness of the icons
C. good appeal to client and family
D. translucency iconicity
E. acceptability to child caretaker

119. In the production and perception of speech sounds which of the following statements reflects an accurate characteristic to distinguish consonants from vowels?

A. Presence of voicing
B. Fundamental frequency
C. Constriction of the vocal tract
D. Oral pressure release
E. Length of duration

120. According to the ASHA Code of Ethics a speech-language pathologist or audiologist must do which of the following?

I. Reveal personal information about clients to legal authorities
II. Provide a guarantee of services
III. Evaluate effectiveness of their services
IV. Refer clients to others to assure highest quality of services

A. I and IV only
B. I, II, and IV only
C. I, III, and IV only
D. II, III, and IV only
E. II and IV only

121. It is appropriate for a speech-language pathologist to provide which of the following services?

A. Conduct newborn hearing screening programs
B. Otoscopic examination and removal of cerumen
C. Assessment and nonmedical management of tinnitus
D. Conduct pure tone air conduction hearing screening
E. Evaluate auditory processing disorders

122. Standards for professional service programs in speech-language pathology require all of the following information in client records EXCEPT

A. referral source and reason for the referral
B. authorization for release of information
C. reports from other professionals
D. documentation of follow-up activities
E. insurance company and record of payment

123. A 4-year-old boy with a repaired bilateral cleft palate exhibits the following characteristics which suggest velopharyngeal incompetency: hypernasality on production of vowels, liquids, and glides; nasal emission on pressure consonants; glottal stops; pharyngeal fricatives; and nasal grimaces. Due to compensatory strategies, his speech is moderately unintelligible. His parents want their son's speech to improve. The most appropriate treatment strategy is

A. exercises to improve velopharyngeal valving
B. articulation therapy targeting all error sounds
C. multifaceted articulation exercises to improve closure and effect correct placement
D. develop articulation training exercises for use by parents at home
E. develop sensory awareness of articulatory placement

124. A clinician has successfully reduced the rate of dysfluencies of a 10-year-old child in the therapy environment. The most appropriate next step should be to

A. dismiss the child from therapy and follow up in 6 months
B. counsel the parents on how to maintain fluency behavior
C. provide play therapy aimed at eliminating the psychological causal factors
D. train carryover activities to promote dysfluency reduction in other environments
E. terminate therapy and provide parents with exercises to continue in home activities

125. Which of the following treatment strategies has been shown to induce fluency in stutterers?

A. Systematic desensitization
B. Delayed auditory feedback
C. Role enactment
D. Personalized fluency control
E. Negative practice

126. J.M. is a 6-year-old girl whose parents are seeking clinical services for her stuttering behaviors. From the evaluation, she is observed to talk very little, but when she does her speech is marked by many syllable and sound repetitions, sound prolongations, and avoidance behaviors. Her parents, who are both professionals, report that they would like J.M to be like her older brother who is intellectually gifted. Because of work responsibilities there is a lack of availability of the parents to J.M. and her brother, but during meals family members are required to talk together at length. In designing a therapy plan for J.M. the clinician should choose which of the following techniques?

A. Environmental manipulation with fluency control
B. Environmental manipulation with psychological therapy

C. Psychological therapy only
D. Environmental manipulation only
E. Fluency control only

127. Variation in treatment practices for stutterers are partially a function of what is perceived as the major causative factor of the problem. A clinician who implements fluency shaping therapy is most probably a proponent of which of the following theories?

A. Biochemical/Physiological theory
B. Genetic theory
C. Neuropsycholinguistic theory
D. Diagnosogenic/Semantogenic theory
E. Neurotic theory

128. A 75-year-old man was diagnosed with severe flaccid dysarthria following a brainstem stroke. Muscular function characterized by reduced range and velocity involving the velum, tongue, lips, and larynx rendered speech severely unintelligible. The most immediate program of rehabilitation should involve

A. modification and strengthening of tone and strength
B. improvement of articulatory precision
C. providing an alternate communication mode
D. enabling the client to respond to targeted goals
E. increasing respiratory function

129. Intervention strategies to improve motor speech disorders involving contrastive stress drills, rate manipulation, and delayed auditory feedback are most useful for

A. modification of resonance
B. modification of phonation
C. modification of respiration
D. modification of prosody
E. modification of strength and tone

130. Mr. Lee, a 69-year-old retired serviceman, sustained a right hemisphere stroke one year ago. Currently he has left hemiparesis, but walks unaided and performs most functions accurately but in a slow and labored manner. His speech is intelligible but lacks emotionality and expression and he unknowingly violates pragmatic rules for conversation. An appropriate intervention goal for Mr. Lee is

A. Mr. Lee will increase attention span
B. In the context of a play, Mr. Lee will assume roles of various characters
C. Mr. Lee will improve fine and gross motor function
D. Mr. Lee will respond appropriately and explain the meaning of jokes
E. Mr. Lee will attend to objects placed in his left visual field

131. Which of the following is NOT an acceptable approach to intervention in dysarthria?

A. Augmentative device
B. Surgery
C. Orthodontal prosthesis
D. Alaryngeal speech
E. Drugs

132. In counseling family members of a client with verbal apraxia which of the following is NOT an appropriate suggestion?

A. Encourage the client to whisper speech
B. Encourage the client to try harder
C. Do not interrupt pauses in the client's speech
D. Encourage the client to use trial and error
E. Expect the client to display automatic behaviors, but to have difficulty with intentional behaviors

133. Which of the following would NOT result in a conductive hearing loss?

A. A teenager regularly attends rock concerts and listens to music through earphones

B. A school-age child is found to have impacted cerumen
C. A preschool child inserts a bead into the ear canal
D. An adult male accident victim has interrupted the ossicular chain
E. A toddler has recurrent bouts of otitis media

134. A hard-of-hearing client reports that in conversation the speech of other individuals is barely audible, yet when they increase their loudness they appear to be shouting. Based on this evidence, the most appropriate diagnostic procedure to be conducted is

A. Short Inventory Sensitivity Index
B. Auditory Brain Stem Response
C. Tone Decay Test
D. Acoustic Reflex Test
E. Békésy Comfortable Loudness Test

135. Which of the following accurately describes the type of hearing loss represented by the accompanying audiogram?

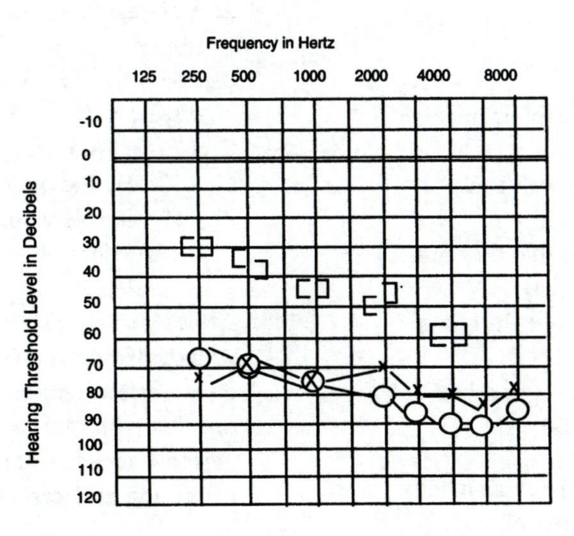

A. Unilateral, severe, conductive
B. Unilateral, severe, sensorineural
C. Bilateral, severe, mixed
D. Bilateral, mild, sensorineural
E. Bilateral, moderate, sensorineural

136. A 70-year-old man is admitted to the hospital following a mild stroke. Staff concerns are that he has lost considerable weight and eats small amounts accompanied by coughing. Which of the following would be the most appropriate recommendation by the speech-language pathologist?

A. Insertion of a nasogastric tube
B. Nothing per oral (npo) status
C. Modified barium swallow study
D. Bedside evaluation of swallowing
E. Oral motor exercise to improve swallowing

137. Which of the following is NOT an appropriate intervention technique for dysphagia patients with pooling in the valleculae?

A. Thermal tactile stimulation
B. Chin tuck
C. Double swallow
D. Oral motor exercises
E. Neck rotation

138. Which of the following clients with hearing loss is an appropriate candidate for a cochlear implant?

A. A 65-year-old man has been diagnosed with presbycusis
B. A 3-year-old boy acquires a profound bilateral sensorineural hearing loss following a bout of rubella
C. A 6-year-old girl has a profound conductive hearing loss
D. A 45-year-old woman is diagnosed with Ménière's disease
E. A 17-year-old girl has otosclerosis

139. Research suggests that parents experience emotional trauma in reaction to the news that their child has an irreversible hearing disability. An effective strategy for easing the shock of bad news is

A. delay delivery of the test results until parents have had a chance to adjust emotionally

B. provide test results gradually over an extended period of time
C. allow parents to observe as the tests are being conducted
D. suggest that parents seek counseling when the test results are provided
E. provide a written report of the test results along with literature about hearing loss

140. Which of the following clients would best benefit from a permanent augmentative communication system?

A. An adult female with voluntary mutism
B. An elderly man with Wernicke's aphasia
C. A college student with moderate dysfluencies
D. A teenager who has mutational falsetto
E. A child who has a profound hearing loss

141. The IEP team for a child with cerebral palsy and mild mental retardation determines that the child can benefit from an assistive communication device. However, the school system has stated that it does not have the funds to provide the child with the required technology. The speech-language pathologist should

A. find an alternative source for acquiring the device
B. inform the parents that they should purchase the device
C. inform the school system that they must provide the device under law
D. encourage the parents to sue the school system
E. request that funds be put in next year's budget and rewrite the IEP

142. A clinician conducts a therapy session with an aphasic client. The objective of the session is 95% accuracy in a cloze exercise using verbal prompts such as "I talk on the ________" which are progressively expanded to other sentences such as "I answer the ________." The client most likely has which of the following?

A. Verbal apraxia
B. Anomia
C. Receptive aphasia
D. Paraphasia
E. Echolalia

143. A speech-language pathologist conducts an evaluation on a 68-year-old woman following the initial onset of a cerebral vascular accident. Results of the testing reveal deficits in both comprehension and language production which are mild to moderate in severity. Based on these results an appropriate first goal of therapy should be to

A. increase motor function
B. increase receptive language skills
C. increase expressive language skills
D. increase functional communication skills
E. enhance spontaneous recovery

144. Melodic Intonation Therapy (MIT) would be most beneficial to which of the following clients

A. a 27-year-old man with traumatic brain injury
B. a 69-year-old woman with Alzheimer's disease
C. a 75-year-old woman with presbycusis
D. a 60-year-old man with Broca's aphasia
E. a 63-year-old woman with right brain dysfunction

145. Speech characteristics of a client diagnosed with dysarthria as a result of Parkinson's disease reflect reduced loudness and stress together with short bursts of speech. An objective measure of the client's aerodynamic and lung capacity may be obtained by

A. oral manometer
B. strain gauge transducer
C. pneumotachygraph
D. nasometer
E. videoendoscopy

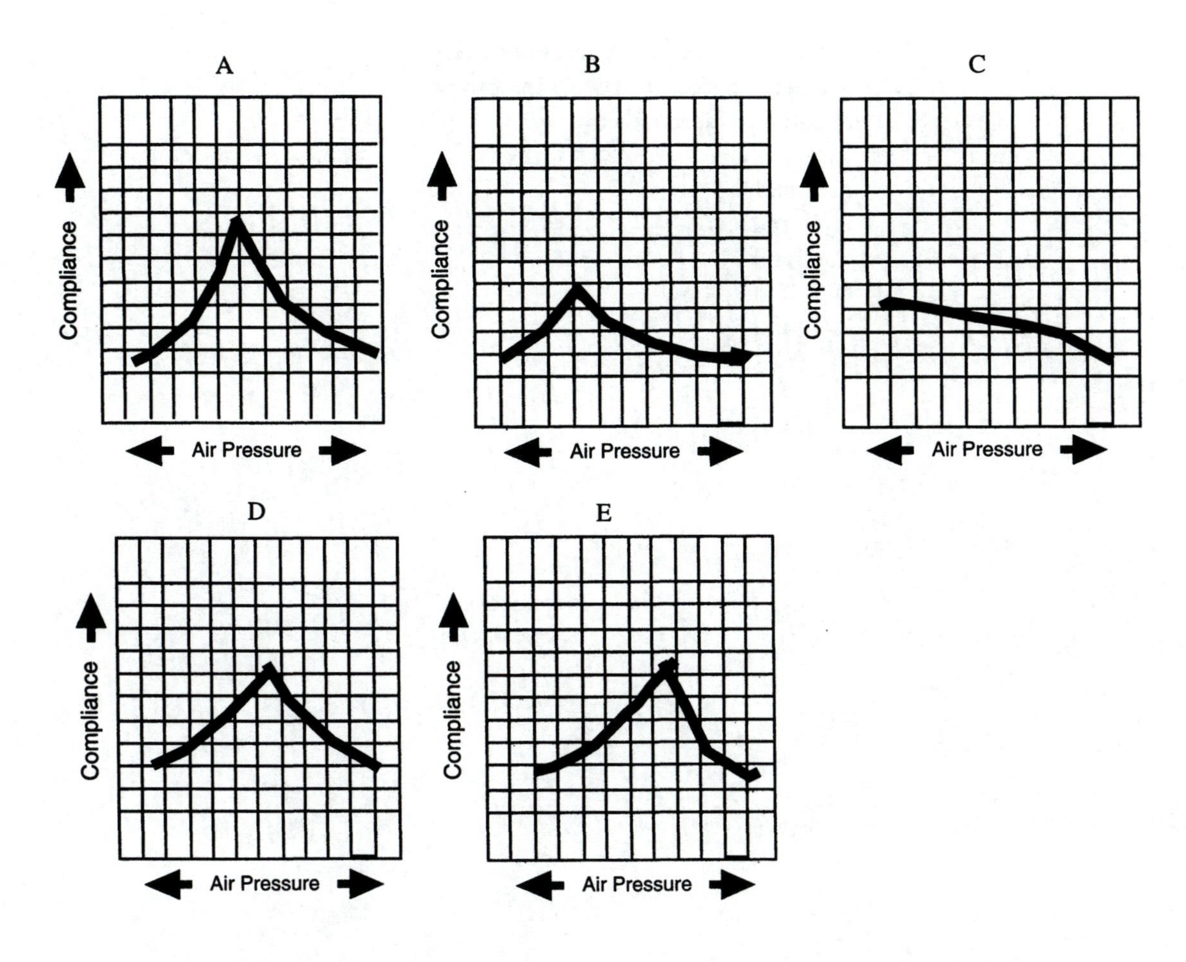

146. Which of the accompanying tympanograms reflects the presence of otitis media?

A. A
B. B
C. C
D. D
E. E

147. The perceptual result of contraction of the cricothyroid muscle is

A. decreased pitch
B. increased pitch
C. increased intensity
D. decreased intensity
E. cessation of phonation

148. During a routine oral examination a clinician observes a high palatal vault along with a relatively short velum and uvula. Which of the following groups of sounds would be expected to be affected?

A. bilabials
B. alveolars
C. stop plosives
D. nasals
E. fricatives

149. The general focus of treatment for a 79-year-old woman with Alzheimer's dementia should be

A. to preserve communication and compensate for loss
B. to provide alternative means for communication
C. to restore communicative function
D. to enable the client to express her needs
E. to make the remaining life as comfortable as possible

150. In the spectrographic analysis of speech, manner and place of articulation can be recognized respectively by

A. F_0 and F_1
B. F_1 and F_2
C. F_0 and F_2
D. F_1 and F_3
E. F_2 and F_3

ANSWER SHEET

CERTIFICATION STATEMENT: (Please write the following statement below. DO NOT PRINT.)
"I hereby agree to the conditions set forth in the Registration Bulletin and certify that I am the person whose name and address appear on this answer sheet."

____

____

____

SIGNATURE________________________________ DATE: ___/___/___

BE SURE EACH MARK IS DARK AND COMPLETELY FILLS THE INTENDED SPACE AS ILLUSTRATED HERE ⬬

1	A B C D E	41	A B C D E	81	A B C D E	121	A B C D E
2	A B C D E	42	A B C D E	82	A B C D E	122	A B C D E
3	A B C D E	43	A B C D E	83	A B C D E	123	A B C D E
4	A B C D E	44	A B C D E	84	A B C D E	124	A B C D E
5	A B C D E	45	A B C D E	85	A B C D E	125	A B C D E
6	A B C D E	46	A B C D E	86	A B C D E	126	A B C D E
7	A B C D E	47	A B C D E	87	A B C D E	127	A B C D E
8	A B C D E	48	A B C D E	88	A B C D E	128	A B C D E
9	A B C D E	49	A B C D E	89	A B C D E	129	A B C D E
10	A B C D E	50	A B C D E	90	A B C D E	130	A B C D E
11	A B C D E	51	A B C D E	91	A B C D E	131	A B C D E
12	A B C D E	52	A B C D E	92	A B C D E	132	A B C D E
13	A B C D E	53	A B C D E	93	A B C D E	133	A B C D E
14	A B C D E	54	A B C D E	94	A B C D E	134	A B C D E
15	A B C D E	55	A B C D E	95	A B C D E	135	A B C D E
16	A B C D E	56	A B C D E	96	A B C D E	136	A B C D E
17	A B C D E	57	A B C D E	97	A B C D E	137	A B C D E
18	A B C D E	58	A B C D E	98	A B C D E	138	A B C D E
19	A B C D E	59	A B C D E	99	A B C D E	139	A B C D E
20	A B C D E	60	A B C D E	100	A B C D E	140	A B C D E
21	A B C D E	61	A B C D E	101	A B C D E	141	A B C D E
22	A B C D E	62	A B C D E	102	A B C D E	142	A B C D E
23	A B C D E	63	A B C D E	103	A B C D E	143	A B C D E
24	A B C D E	64	A B C D E	104	A B C D E	144	A B C D E
25	A B C D E	65	A B C D E	105	A B C D E	145	A B C D E
26	A B C D E	66	A B C D E	106	A B C D E	146	A B C D E
27	A B C D E	67	A B C D E	107	A B C D E	147	A B C D E
28	A B C D E	68	A B C D E	108	A B C D E	148	A B C D E
29	A B C D E	69	A B C D E	109	A B C D E	149	A B C D E
30	A B C D E	70	A B C D E	110	A B C D E	150	A B C D E
31	A B C D E	71	A B C D E	111	A B C D E	151	A B C D E
32	A B C D E	72	A B C D E	112	A B C D E	152	A B C D E
33	A B C D E	73	A B C D E	113	A B C D E	153	A B C D E
34	A B C D E	74	A B C D E	114	A B C D E	154	A B C D E
35	A B C D E	75	A B C D E	115	A B C D E	155	A B C D E
36	A B C D E	76	A B C D E	116	A B C D E	156	A B C D E
37	A B C D E	77	A B C D E	117	A B C D E	157	A B C D E
38	A B C D E	78	A B C D E	118	A B C D E	158	A B C D E
39	A B C D E	79	A B C D E	119	A B C D E	159	A B C D E
40	A B C D E	80	A B C D E	120	A B C D E	160	A B C D E

PRACTICE TEST CONVERSION CHART*

**Based on approximate values. Values change for each administration of the Praxis.*

Number Right	Scaled Score	Number Right	Scaled Score	Number Right	Scaled Score
0	250				
1	250	50	380	100	640
2	250	51	390	101	640
3	250	52	390	102	650
4	250	53	400	103	660
		54	400	104	660
5	250				
6	250	55	410	105	670
7	250	56	410	106	670
8	250	57	420	107	680
9	250	58	420	108	680
		59	430	109	690
10	250				
11	250	60	430	110	690
12	250	61	440	111	700
13	250	62	440	112	700
14	250	63	450	113	710
		64	450	114	720
15	250				
16	250	65	460	115	720
17	250	66	460	116	730
18	250	67	470	117	730
19	250	68	480	118	740
		69	480	119	740
20	250				
21	250	70	490	120	750
22	250	71	490	121	750
23	250	72	500	122	760
24	250	73	500	123	760
		74	510	124	770
25	250				
26	260	75	510	125	770
27	260	76	520	126	780
28	270	77	520	127	780
29	270	78	530	128	790
		79	530	129	790
30	280				
31	280	80	540	130	800
32	290	81	540	131	800
33	290	82	550	132	810
34	300	83	550	133	810
		84	560	134	829
35	300				
36	310	85	560	135	830
37	310	86	570	136	830
38	320	87	570	137	840
39	320	88	580	138	840
		89	580	139	850
40	330				
41	330	90	590	140	850
42	340	91	600	141	860
43	340	92	600	142	860
44	350	93	610	143	870
		94	610	144	870
45	350				
46	360	95	620	145	880
47	370	96	620	146	880
48	370	97	630	147	890
49	380	98	630	148	890
		99	640	149/150	900

APPENDIX

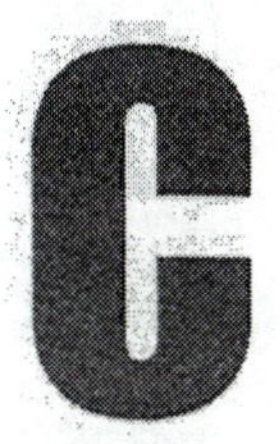

ANSWERS AND EXPLANATIONS FOR THE PRACTICE TEST

PRAXIS—SPEECH-LANGUAGE PATHOLOGY

Time—120 minutes
150 Questions

1. **Answer: C.**
   Reliability is the measurement of consistency across trials.
2. **Answer: A.**
   Effectiveness is measured by reviewing changes or lack of change in the desired behaviors.
3. **Answer: A.**
   An ordinal scale presents options in ordered sequence.
4. **Answer: B.**
   In a Single Group Time Series Design one subject group is observed several times before and after treatment.
5. **Answer: A.**
   Short-term goals of therapy relate to daily or weekly activities and are not a part of the diagnostic report.
6. **Answer: E.**
   The diagnostic report must be precise and objective without speculation and judgment about the child's parent.
7. **Answer: B.**
   In the presence of a genetic history of stuttering parent counseling and intervention are always recommended.
8. **Answer: C.**
   The critical age hypothesis posits that there is a crucial time period for language learning which requires human verbal interaction.
9. **Answer: C.**
   Dialects are not speech disorders, therefore qualified clinicians may provide elective services only by request of the individual.
10. **Answer: C.**
    These are typical initial substitutions for sounds developed after 3 years of age.
11. **Answer: E.**
    Apraxia is a disorder of motor planning characterized by impairment of volitional speech.
12. **Answer: D.**
    D represents the only true statement which is not judgmental.
13. **Answer: D.**
    According to Piaget, the development of object permanence and causality are critical to language development. These are acquired in the sensorimotor and preoperational stages.
14. **Answer: B.**
    A baseline is a measured rate of responding in the absence of treatment.
15. **Answer: A.**
    Formant frequencies correspond to front-back and high-low tongue position for the production of vowels.
16. **Answer: E.**
    Comparison of the potential effects of each option reveals that the most negative effect is rendered by inappropriate stress.
17. **Answer: B.**
    A 51-year-old man is the best candidate because of age, disability condition, intact cognitive ability, and language.
18. **Answer: A.**
    Cessation of babbling is an indicator of deafness because speech develops when babbling is shaped and reinforced.
19. **Answer: D.**
    The child is able to produce /s/, but the rules for its usage as well as usage of /sh/ are simplified.

20. **Answer: E.**
The action of yawning inhibits vocal constriction and relieves vocal fold tension; thus it is most useful in vocal hyperfunction.
21. **Answer: D.**
Articulatory distortions involving manner and place are often heard as less severe than phonemic omissions.
22. **Answer: A.**
All characteristics can be found in both groups except normal to high intelligence.
23. **Answer: D.**
Inter-rater reliability is the indicator of consistency in scoring by two or more judges.
24. **Answer: B.**
A reinforcer is a reward that increases a behavior. Verbal praise is a social reinforcer that is a type of secondary reinforcer.
25. **Answer: C.**
Appropriate use in the natural environment is the definition of behavior maintenance.
26. **Answer: A.**
A probe is a procedure to assess carryover.
27. **Answer: D.**
Shaping involves successive reinforcements of elements of a target response.
28. **Answer: D.**
All are features of African-American English except omission of articles.
29. **Answer: B.**
The clinician reinforces an alternative behavior as a method to increase a desired response.
30. **Answer: D.**
Although individual scores can vary, unbiased tests do not exhibit a pattern of scoring for a given population.
31. **Answer: D.**
All are characteristics of language development in mentally retarded children except these children do not catch up to their peers.
32. **Answer: D.**
Standard English is the only variety (dialect) that is appropriate for writing. Although it is preferred for social advancement, other varieties are not considered "incorrect."
33. **Answer: B.**
This test item requires a child to understand the distinctions between semantic markers, or pronouns such as her, him, them, it.
34. **Answer: D.**
During the holophrastic or one word stage, one word represents a more complex sentence structure.
35. **Answer: C.**
In the process of language development children's utterances are predictable applications of regular rules to linguistic irregularities. "Goed" is a predictable generalization for past tense -ed.
36. **Answer: A.**
Ataxia, a disorder characterized by uncoordinated movements, is the result of injury to the cerebellum which is responsible for the smoothly coordinated movements of muscles.
37. **Answer: B.**
Treatment methods must be derived from sound theory and proven effective by research.
38. **Answer: C.**
Most test instruments are validated in the norming process; therefore, clinicians do not validate instruments during diagnosis.

39. **Answer: E.**
To produce a cognitive change the child must first be able to perceive differences between the error and target sounds; therefore discrimination of error and target sounds should be the initial goal.
40. **Answer: E.**
Because the articulatory mechanism is highly adaptable, absence of dentition has little effect.
41. **Answer: E.**
Absence of grammatical morphemes, unstressed syllable omission, final consonant omission, and cluster simplification may be features of African-American Dialect or language disorder. However, limited vocabulary, stopping, gliding, and decreased intelligibility suggest language disorder inclusive of phonological disorder.
42. **Answer: C.**
To sample emerging phonemes, an age equivalency score must be derived. Phonological analysis does not generate an age equivalency score.
43. **Answer: A.**
The Kahn-Lewis Phonological Analysis is designed to be used with the Goldman-Fristoe Test of Articulation to provide a method of examining phonological processes.
44. **Answer: B.**
Phonological disorders are functional disturbances in speech perception and production related to the phonology component of language.
45. **Answer: B.**
Tongue thrust is a forward motion of the tongue during articulation of sounds requiring static frontal placement such as /s/ or /z/.
46. **Answer: A.**
Specific language impairments occur without cognitive or sensory deficits.
47. **Answer: C.**
Metaphonological ability involves tasks such as rhyming and syllabification which are necessary for reading achievement.
48. **Answer: D.**
The physical context is ultimately important in selecting augmentative and alternative communication systems.
49. **Answer: C.**
Client records may be released only with the written consent of the client or guardian.
50. **Answer: A.**
Transformational rules dictate the positioning of auxiliaries to change a declarative sentence to an interrogative as in "It is raining" to "Is it raining?"
51. **Answer: C.**
Assessment of oral-motor function should be undertaken prior to treatment as well as in the first stage of diagnosis.
52. **Answer: E.**
In-class word substitutions are made when two words share semantic properties.
53. **Answer: C.**
Derivational morphemes conjoin with other morphemes and create a new word often in a different grammatical class.
54. **Answer: B.**
Metathesis is a phonological rule that reorders or transposes sounds.
55. **Answer: D.**
A mass that prevents complete vocal fold closure or adds to thickness will result in changes in vocal

quality. Hyponasality is a disorder of resonance.

56. **Answer: C.**
Pragmatic rules relate to linguistic aspects of communication performance. Eye behavior and gestures are nonlinguistic elements.
57. **Answer: C.**
Metalinguistic ability involves the use of language as a tool for communication such as jokes, sarcasm, and idioms.
58. **Answer: C.**
In an indirect speech act the surface structure (e.g., an interrogative) is used for a different intention (e.g., a request). "Can you pass the salt?" is not a question about the listener's capability, but a request for an action.
59. **Answer: C.**
Least restrictive environment assures education with nondisabled economically disadvantaged children.
60. **Answer: D.**
Part H of P.L. 99-457 requires the development of an Individualized Family Service Plan for at risk children from birth to 2.11 years.
61. **Answer: A.**
Mean Length of Utterance is calculated using a language sample and formula and then computed to expected outcomes per age level. Other choices are norm-referenced diagnostic instruments.
62. **Answer: D.**
Designation of intellectual disabilities begins at 2 standard deviations below the mean; thus an IQ of 68 would be designated as mild.
63. **Answer: D.**
Biological and environmental factors separately and interactively affect treatment outcomes. The best determinant of outcome is the combined number of risk factors rather than any single factor.
64. **Answer: A.**
Since specific language disability is not associated with other deficits the only choice related specifically to language is limited use of vocabulary and grammatical morphemes.
65. **Answer: B.**
Following traumatic brain injury, all of the characteristics listed may occur. Each is summarized in one answer choice which is impairment of attention, perception, and memory.
66. **Answer: C.**
A developmental study compares populations across the age spectrum.
67. **Answer: D.**
A developmental study compares populations across the age spectrum.
68. **Answer: B.**
In an experimental study the dependent variable is the effect or outcome of the stimulus; thus a change in the sucking response is the outcome of changing auditory stimuli.
69. **Answer: A.**
The symptoms described are indicative of cluttering dysfluency.
70. **Answer: E.**
The criterion for dismissal is based on achievement of objectives rather than environmental influences.
71. **Answer: D.**
A client may be able to imitate, a subcognitive ability indicating phonetic perception. However, meaningful awareness, discrimination, and production of the sound at a phonological level may not be present.

72. **Answer: C.**
Breathiness is the acoustic effect when excessive air escapes during phonation as a result of incomplete closure of the vocal folds.
73. **Answer: E.**
The most likely cause of Joseph's hoarseness is vocal nodules which occur bilaterally at the junction of the anterior and middle thirds where vocal folds strike most vigorously.
74. **Answer: C.**
Autism is a social disorder based on a failure to establish communicative relationships with others.
75. **Answer: A.**
If velopharyngeal closure cannot be made, there is both nasal and oral escape and the result is hypernasality.
76. **Answer: B.**
A papilloma, which is similar to a wart, is a benign neoplasm of childhood.
77. **Answer: D.**
Sound is produced when air is forced through the constriction at the pharyngeo-esophageal segment which is the juncture between the pharynx and esophagus.
78. **Answer: D.**
The routine voice examination includes evaluation of vocal quality, resonance, pitch, and intensity.
79. **Answer: C.**
Before more aggressive therapies are undertaken, collaboration with a psychologist will help to establish and address the cause of the vocal disorder.
80. **Answer: A.**
Videofluorography allows the viewing of structural movements in action.
81. **Answer: B.**
Omission of final consonants is the most frequent articulatory pattern of hearing-impaired individuals.
82. **Answer: B.**
A criterion-referenced instrument compares client performance to a preset score.
83. **Answer: D.**
A prognosis is a prediction of a client performance after treatment.
84. **Answer: B.**
African-American English is a cultural variety of English with distinct features based on predictable language changes and rules for its usage.
85. **Answer: B.**
A well-written diagnostic report is fully descriptive so as to support the recommendations.
86. **Answer: B.**
A regional or foreign accent derives from linguistic influences manifested basically in pronunciation and syllabification.
87. **Answer: B.**
A creole is a language derived from mixing of two languages that eventually becomes the language of a specific community.
88. **Answer: B.**
Any variety of a language is known as a dialect. Although dialect features differ from the standard, these features are not errors.
89. **Answer: C.**
Most of the choices would be unethical or untenable. The test should be modified appropriately to eliminate the bias against the client.
90. **Answer: A.**
The client's symptoms suggest neurological involvement and are

symptoms which accompany aphasia.

91. **Answer: C.**
A Mean Length of Utterance of 4.5 is expected for a child of 4 years of age.

92. **Answer: A.**
Although ease of administration of tests in terms of timing may be a concern of clinicians with a heavy case load, the highest value of the profession is concern for the client.

93. **Answer: B.**
The tests given do not include a measure of functional ability to examine everyday life skills.

94. **Answer: C.**
A major indicator of right hemisphere dysfunction is left side neglect, which is not observed in left hemisphere lesions.

95. **Answer: C.**
The Rancho Los Amigos rating scale for traumatic brain injury has 8 levels ranging from unresponsive to fully recovered. A level IV rating is moderate in severity.

96. **Answer: D.**
The Scales of Cognitive Ability for Traumatic Brain Injury examine psychological abilities that are symptoms of generalized closed head injury.

97. **Answer: C.**
The Communication Abilities in Daily Living (CADL) is a measure of ability to function independently in the environment.

98. **Answer: B.**
The McDonald Deep Test of Articulation examines error phonemes in various phonetic environments as they release into or terminate from other sounds.

99. **Answer: C.**
Characteristics of verbal apraxia include periods of well-articulated speech, especially on automatic tasks. Errors of phonological disorders are consistent across contexts.

100. **Answer: B.**
Gliding involves substitution of a glide for a liquid as in w/l, while cluster reduction involves elimination of one element of a blend as in t/tr.

101. **Answer: D.**
Dysarthria is a disorder that results from muscular impairment. Errors are consistent and predictable.

102. **Answer: C.**
Apraxia is a disorder of motor planning rather than muscle weakness.

103. **Answer: A.**
Since apraxia is not a disorder of muscle weakness the oral examination appears normal. However, as a disorder of motor planning, errors are unpredictable and become more severe as the nature of the task increases in complexity.

104. **Answer: C.**
Since apraxia is a disorder of motor planning, precise timing of the sounds may be affected, producing correct sounds out of sequence.

105. **Answer: A.**
Overly adducted vocal folds require more air pressure from the lungs to affect vibration. This in turn produces increased intensity.

106. **Answer: C.**
The s/z ratio is a reflection of the completeness of closure of the vocal folds. Organic voice disorders involving vocal fold masses

reflect incomplete closure with an s/z ratio higher than 1.0.

107. **Answer: A.**
Modification of behavioral and environmental conditions is essential to improvement of voice disorders of both organic and nonorganic origin.

108. **Answer: B.**
Videoendoscopy is the only method that allows visual inspection of movement to be recorded on videotape.

109. **Answer: C.**
Five-year-olds exhibit normal dysfluencies which are whole word repetitions.

110. **Answer: B.**
The adaptation effect is a measure of dysfluency assessing consistency of dysfluent behavior over 3 trials on the same words.

111. **Answer: B.**
The goal of assessment for an augmentative device is to accurately detail a client's level of functioning across several domains to determine if an augmentative device is appropriate.

112. **Answer: A.**
The Stocker Probe Technique allows observation of dysfluency in relationship to increasing communicative demands.

113. **Answer: B.**
Flatulence would be an indicator of lower gastrointestinal problems rather than swallowing.

114. **Answer: D.**
A modified barium swallow procedure would be used to confirm the presence of aspiration suspected from results of the bedside examination.

115. **Answer: C.**
Food comes in contact with the nasopharynx during the pharyngeal stage of swallowing.

116. **Answer: B.**
Videofiberoptic endoscopy allows inspection of the larynx before and after swallowing to detect the presence of food in the larynx.

117. **Answer: A.**
A major concern of a 16-year-old might be the speed of the device in formulating communication responses.

118. **Answer: A.**
A symbol will be acceptable to a child if it is structured to be simple, easy to learn, and distinguished from others.

119. **Answer: C.**
Consonants are created by forming a major constriction of the vocal tract, while in the production of vowels airflow is relatively unrestricted.

120. **Answer: C.**
A speech-language pathologist or audiologist is prohibited from providing a guarantee of services.

121. **Answer: D.**
It is within the scope of practice of speech-language pathologists to provide audiological screenings.

122. **Answer: E.**
Financial records are not a requisite part of the client's folder.

123. **Answer: C.**
Exercises to improve velopharyngeal valving have not proven effective; however, there is evidence that well-developed articulation strategies may influence closure.

124. **Answer: D.**
Prior to dismissal from therapy

the clinician should ensure carry-over from therapy to the living environment.

125. **Answer: B.**
Delayed auditory feedback has been shown to induce fluency by altering the stutterer's ability to simultaneously monitor speech, thus eliminating the anticipation of stuttering.

126. **Answer: A.**
The child's speech contains many stuttering characteristics that are probably being maintained by the home environment, thus both environment and fluency should be addressed.

127. **Answer: C.**
Neuropsycholinguistic theories posit that there is a disruption between the linguistic system and the signal system that must converge to create the articulation programming for fluent speech. Fluency shaping is aimed at providing feedback for self monitoring of speech.

128. **Answer: D.**
Enabling the client to respond to targeted goals is the most basic skill, which may include counseling and education about the disorder prior to specific drill and exercise.

129. **Answer: D.**
Modification of prosody—that is, rhythm, stress, and intonation—should focus on stress drills and altering the rate of speech.

130. **Answer: B.**
Acting as all characters in a play will enable the client to increase emotionality and expression and practice pragmatic rules of conversation. Other options do not address the specific communication disabilities of the client.

131. **Answer: D.**
Alaryngeal speech is restricted to cases of laryngectomy.

132. **Answer: B.**
Attempts by apraxic clients to try harder produces more errors.

133. **Answer: A.**
Recent findings are that prolonged exposure to loud noise damages auditory hair cells resulting in sensorineural hearing loss.

134. **Answer: A.**
The symptoms of the client suggest the phenomenon of recruitment, which is diagnosed by the Short Inventory Sensitivity Index (SISI).

135. **Answer: C.**
There is a greater loss for air conduction than bone conduction in both ears, with a gap larger than 10 dB (mixed) and both are abnormal. ANSI standard for severe hearing loss is 66 to 95 dB.

136. **Answer: D.**
A bedside swallow examination should be conducted prior to any decisions or actions.

137. **Answer: A.**
Postural techniques such as chin tuck are useful in preventing and eliminating residue by temporarily altering the anatomical configuration of the pharynx.

138. **Answer: B.**
Cochlear implants are not effective for conductive hearing losses, but restore nerve conduction from the cochlea that has been caused by sensorineural hearing loss.

139. **Answer: C.**
Allowing parents to observe, even to participate in the hearing evaluation, prepares them to be more receptive to the results when given.

140. **Answer: E.**
An augmentative/alternative communication device is most appropriate for individuals who are not amenable to conventional methods of rehabilitation.

141. **Answer: C.**
Under the Individuals with Disabilities Education Act (IDEA), school systems cannot refuse to provide assistive technology if a determination is made by an IEP team.

142. **Answer: B.**
A client with anomia has difficulty with confrontation naming. A cloze procedure altering prompts that require the same word response is appropriate treatment.

143. **Answer: B.**
The extent of language recovery is related to the degree to which receptive language is impaired. A logical first goal is to increase receptive language skills.

144. **Answer: D.**
Melodic Intonation Therapy (MIT) is most effective for highly motivated patients with a unilateral left hemisphere lesion.

145. **Answer: C.**
The most accepted instrument for measuring volume rate of airflow is pneumotachygraphy, which measures both ingressive and egressive airflow.

146. **Answer: C.**
The presence of fluid in the middle ear produces negative pressure as well as increased mass, resulting in a Type C or flat tympanogram.

147. **Answer: B.**
As the cricothyroid muscle contracts the thyroid cartilage tilts forward, thus increasing the length of the vocal folds and increasing pitch.

148. **Answer: C.**
A high palatal arch with soft tissue insufficiency would result in inadequate velopharyngeal closure, which is necessary for interoral pressure for stop plosives.

149. **Answer: A.**
Because dementia is a progressive condition involving loss of cognitive function, the goal of treatment should be to preserve present communicative abilities and compensate for those which have been lost.

150. **Answer: B.**
F_0, F_2, and F_3 relate to formant bands which are spectrographic displays of energy in a speech sound related to vocal tract configurations. The shifts of F_1 reflect the manner of articulation and the shifts in F_2 reflect place of articulation.

APPENDIX

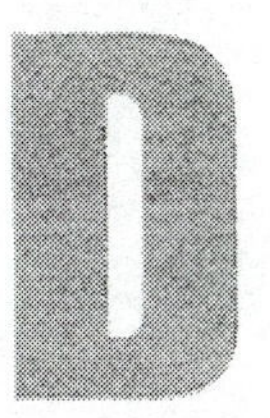

DIAGNOSTIC INDICATORS

1. You did not complete all questions in the examination within the designated time.

   Use the Praxis Computer Practice Module to increase your timing. Refer to Unit 8 of this book.

2. You answered fewer than 95 questions correctly.

   Review the examination, taking note of your areas of weakness, e.g., course areas, types of questions. Review course content and practice with the Praxis Computer Practice Module to improve your knowledge in these areas.

3. Many of the questions were unknown to you.

   Update your knowledge of the field through self study. Use the computer-aided instruction unit of the Praxis Computer Practice Module.

4. You recognized the correct answers after you scored the examination, but during the actual test, you got them wrong.

   Your problem may be complex, ranging from poor judgment, or lack of test-taking skills to test anxiety. Review each unit of this book. Use the test-taking skills and cognitive skills exercises of the Praxis Computer Practice Module.

5. You scored well on the Practice Examination, but not as well on the actual Praxis.

   You may be experiencing test anxiety. Refer to Unit 6.

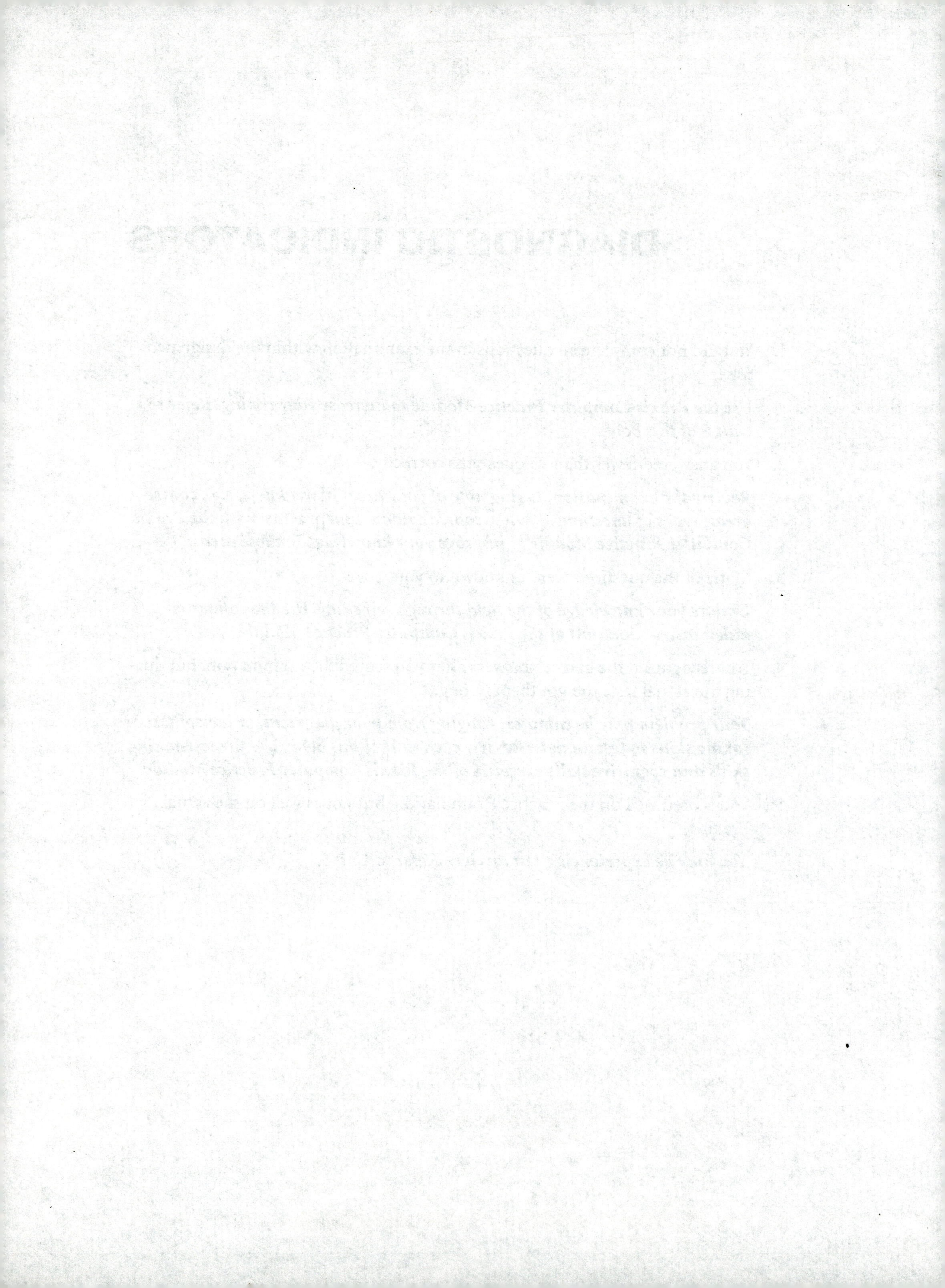